Atlas of
Nuclear Imaging
in Sports Medicine

Atlas of
Nuclear
Imaging
in Sports
Medicine

Robert Cooper
Stephen Allwright
Jock Anderson

The **McGraw·Hill** Companies

Sydney New York San Francisco Auckland
Bangkok Bogotá Caracas Hong Kong
Kuala Lumpur Lisbon London Madrid
Mexico City Milan New Delhi San Juan
Seoul Singapore Taipei Toronto

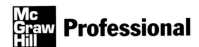

Notice

Medicine is an ever-changing science. As new research and clinical experience broaden our knowledge, changes in treatment and drug therapy are required. The editors and the publisher of this work have checked with sources believed to be reliable in their efforts to provide information that is complete and generally in accord with the standards accepted at the time of publication. However, in view of the possibility of human error or changes in medical sciences, neither the editors, nor the publisher, nor any other party who has been involved in the preparation or publication of this work warrants that the information contained herein is in every respect accurate or complete. Readers are encouraged to confirm the information contained herein with other sources. For example, and in particular, readers are advised to check the product information sheet included in the package of each drug they plan to administer to be certain that the information contained in this book is accurate and that changes have not been made in the recommended dose or in the contraindications for administration. This recommendation is of particular importance in connection with new or infrequently used drugs.

National Library of Australia Cataloguing-in-Publication data:

Cooper, Robert, 1946–.
Atlas of nuclear imaging in sports medicine.

Includes index.
ISBN 0 074 71088 5.
1. Sports injuries—Imaging—Atlases. 2. Sports injuries—Diagnosis. 3. Diagnostic imaging—Atlases. 4. Sports medicine—Atlases.
I. Anderson, Ian F., 1941–. II. Allwright, Stephen, 1954–. III. Title.

617.1027

Published in Australia by
McGraw-Hill Australia Pty Ltd
Level 2, 82 Waterloo Road, North Ryde, NSW 2113
Publishing Manager: Meiling Voon
Production Editor: Rosemary McDonald
Editor: Joy Window
Proofreader: Tim Learner
Indexer: Diane Harriman
Design (interior and cover): Jan Schmoeger/Designpoint
Image preparation: Peter Freeman, Freedom Graphics
Typeset in 10/12 pt Franklin Gothic by Jan Schmoeger/Designpoint
Printed on 80 gsm matt art by Pantech Ltd, Hong Kong.

The McGraw-Hill Companies

Foreword

The majority of people in the world engage in athletic activities at some point in their lives. As a counterbalance to all of the positive aspects of that, is the predictable and inevitable occurrence of sport injuries. The specialised nature of these injuries, both diagnostically and therapeutically, has led to the establishment of Sports Medicine as a recognized specialty area encompassing the efforts of orthopaedic surgeons, radiologists and nuclear medicine specialists among others.

Early accurate diagnosis is the key to successful management of patients with sports injuries. Drs. Cooper, Allwright and Anderson have done a brilliant job in their new book *Atlas of Nuclear Imaging in Sports Medicine* in putting together a comprehensive scintigraphic approach to the diagnosis of sports injuries. Anyone involved in the care of patients with these injuries will welcome this book and its logical, accessible format.

For the nuclear medicine specialist, the technical approaches are nicely summarised in the first chapter. The authors point out the importance of Single Photon Emission Computed Tomography (SPECT) and such special methods as 3-phase scintigraphy. A truly valuable aspect of the *Atlas of Nuclear Imaging in Sports Medicine* is the inclusion of technical tips for each anatomic imaging site. The ability to tailor the skeletal scintigram to both the anatomic structures being imaged and to the most likely conditions ensures optimum sensitivity and specificity. This is a unique feature of the *Atlas of Nuclear Imaging in Sports Medicine* not found in general textbooks of nuclear medicine.

The second chapter presents the conceptual basis for using nuclear skeletal scintigraphy in the diagnosis of sports injuries. In parallel with the discussion of underlying pathophysiology of skeletal and soft tissue injuries, the authors clearly outline the advantages of scintigraphy, its limitations and how it fits into an overall diagnostic approach that may require the use of multiple imaging modalities. This is refreshing from the standpoint that proponents of one imaging modality or another frequently try to overstate the utility of their particular interest. Drs. Cooper, Allwright and Anderson, to their credit, do not do this but provide appropriate perspective for the reader.

The greatest strength of the *Atlas of Nuclear Imaging in Sports Medicine* is its comprehensiveness in covering sports injuries by both type of injury and location. Thus, the same basic kind of injury may take on quite different scintigraphic appearances in different anatomic sites and the presentation of a few examples, as found in most general textbooks of nuclear medicine, in no way presents the reader with a full range of examples. Further, the authors have the benefit of drawing their illustrative material from their substantial clinical experiences garnered from years of practice making this book a near definitive collection of sports injuries and superior to any existing work.

The *Atlas of Nuclear Imaging in Sports Medicine* should be of interest to orthopaedic surgeons specialising in sports medicine and to radiologists and nuclear medicine specialists who encounter sports injuries in their practices. In fact, for diagnostic imaging specialists, the ability to build and sustain a practice in a given subspecialty area is often determined by the special value they are able to deliver in the care of patients. Radiologists and nuclear medicine physicians who take advantage of the information provided in this book will be well served in building significant practices related to sports medicine.

Finally, speaking from my own experience as a writer and author, it is an extraordinary undertaking to produce a book of any kind. The hours required and the attention to detail are daunting. Since all physicians depend on knowledge as the basis of their practices, we must voice our gratitude to peers and colleagues who are willing to undertake the task of organising information to our collective benefit. I congratulate and thank Drs. Cooper, Allwright and Anderson for their undertaking and for delivering such an outstanding book to the benefit of physicians and their patients who are confronting sports medicine injuries.

James H. Thrall, M.D.
Chairman, Department of Radiology
Massachusetts General Hospital
Professor of Radiology,
Harvard Medical School

Contents

Preface

Sport, both elite and recreational, plays an important role in society in recent times. An increasing number of people participate more often, and frequently to levels of training more complex and demanding than before. Physicians encourage the benefits of increased exercise. Along with all the benefits which accrue from this increased physical activity comes an increasing incidence of injuries. Some of these injuries are due to direct trauma such as in contact sports. Others, however, are due to overuse injuries and these frequently occur during training periods.

Accompanying this growth in sports and physical activity has been the evolution of the specialty of sports medicine. Nuclear medicine has grown and evolved with sports medicine. It not only has helped in the diagnosing of sports injuries, but also has aided in our understanding of the pathophysiology of many conditions.

The role of nuclear medicine has changed over the years and has also been altered by the emergence of other technologies now in common clinical usage. These include ultrasound, CT and MRI. Nuclear medicine, however, still plays a large and frequently pivotal role. This atlas is designed to demonstrate the spectrum of appearances of the many conditions seen in sports medicine, rather than a single 'typical' case. The gamut of cases provides a practical reference for students and practitioners of both sports medicine and nuclear medicine.

To facilitate easy reference, the atlas is set out anatomically. This means that different conditions in the same anatomic region, which may present in similar clinical ways, are grouped together. The introductory chapters cover the pathologies encountered in sports medicine, the science of nuclear medicine and the basic concepts involved in tailoring the nuclear medicine study to achieve optimal sports medicine imaging and clinically useful results. An understanding of the basic pathophysiology aids scan interpretation and will help nuclear medicine grow with the continuing changes in sports medicine.

Acknowledgments

The authors wish to sincerely thank a number of people who have helped in the production of this book. In particular, we would like to acknowledge the contribution of the Nuclear Medicine Technologists at the North Shore Nuclear Medicine Department at the Mater Misericordiae Hospital, North Sydney and at Dee Why Nuclear Medicine who have worked with us over the years, including Anne Moase, David Raffles, John Howard, Sue King, Sally Raymond, Carol Goodier and Sue Lazarus. Their attention to detail and consistent desire to obtain the best possible quality study have been invaluable. Our secretarial staff have also been a great help and in particular we wish to thank Rae Henderson for clerical assistance. Stame George's computer assistance was greatly appreciated.

We are indebted to the staff of the North Sydney Orthopaedic and Sports Medicine Centre and the Narrabeen Sports Medicine Centre. These two groups headed by Dr Ken Crichton and Dr Stuart Watson have been very supportive for many years and have contributed greatly to our understanding of Sports Medicine.

We also wish to thank David McHarg, John Burke and Ruth Highet for the images they kindly provided. These are acknowledged in the captions to the images. David McHarg's reviews of the manuscript were most helpful. In the production phase, special thanks are also conveyed to Peter Freeman for his expert help in image preparation and Jan Schmoeger for his skill in layout and design.

Finally and most importantly we thank our wives, Ligita and Tracey, and our families for their forbearance, inspiration and encouragement to persist whenever our enthusiasm for the task waned.

1 Technical considerations

With the increasing community interest in physical fitness and sport comes the growing demand for a medical infrastructure with special skills in the diagnosis and management of musculoskeletal injury. These skills are many and varied and are supplied by a team of professionals. The team includes sports physicians, orthopaedic surgeons, physiotherapists, podiatrists, sports scientists, dieticians and sports psychologists. The imaging specialist is also a pivotal member of this team. It is important to remember that appropriate treatment relies on an initial accurate diagnosis.

An understanding of the basic pathological process that occurs with tissue injury is the key to the selection of the appropriate imaging pathway. Each imaging method creates an image using different technology and different information is produced. All methods have their strengths and weaknesses and tend to be used in sequence rather than in isolation, building up information until the changes are clearly anatomically identified and characterised.

Plain radiology is the starting point of almost all protocols and very often is the only imaging method required if the clinically suspected change, such as a fracture, is shown. If the plain films are normal and clinical suspicion persists, other imaging methods are then used. In this situation, a bone scan may show an area of abnormality within bone that may be diagnostic or can be further defined and characterised by CT or perhaps MRI. If the abnormality is thought to be soft tissue, then ultrasound or MRI may enable a diagnosis to be made.

It is also important to remember that imaging depends on the skill and knowledge of the operator. Knowledge of sports medicine and of the biomechanics of the injury contribute significantly to the quality and accuracy of the imaging report. Ultrasound, in particular, is operator-dependent.

The bone scan

The bone scan has been used in sports medicine since its inception.

Radiopharmaceuticals

Technetium phosphate agents, methylene diphosphonate (MDP) or hydroxymethylene diphosphonate (HMDP), are the commonest agents used in bone scanning. Despite their use for 20 years the mechanism of uptake remains debatable. It is known that the uptake of these radio-pharmaceuticals is dependent on blood flow and the extraction efficiency of a particular tissue. The relationship between blood flow and uptake is not linear with the uptake being less than the proportional increase in blood flow.

The flow and early blood pool images demonstrate the blood flow to the area of interest (see *The three-phase bone scan* below). Some conditions will show increased flow, others normal flow and less commonly reduced or absent flow. This information is helpful in the specificity of diagnosis.

The extraction efficiency is the other determinant of the degree of uptake. This has been shown to be a function of:

- the calcium content of tissues;
- the nature of the calcium/phosphate complexes;
- the nature of the bone matrix;
- the metabolic activity of the bone;
- the bone surface area exposed to extracellular fluid and blood.

Uptake can occur in extraosseous sites, where it is also related to blood flow and extraction efficiency. Altered calcium metabolism in muscle can result in uptake in both skeletal and cardiac muscle following injury.

A simple but useful generalisation is that the uptake depends on the blood flow and the metabolic activity of bone. So, with bone scans, we rely on the increase in metabolic activity caused by the bone's response to a particular insult such as fracture, neoplasm or infection. We image the response to insult rather than the actual insult, this response being a very sensitive indicator of bone pathology.

The gamma camera

The radiopharmaceutical localises in both normal and abnormal tissues and gamma rays are emitted in all directions. The gamma rays that are used to form the image are collimated, so that only the rays perpendicular to the camera face contribute to the image. These photons pass into a crystal where they react to produce a light flash. The light flash is then localised by a system of photomultiplier tubes, producing an X and Y pulse. In addition, the intensity of the light flash is measured, producing a Z pulse. These pulses are then electronically transmitted to a computer. Multiple counts are collected to build up an image.

Collimator

The majority of bone imaging is performed with a high-resolution parallel hole collimator. This gives a high resolution two-dimensional image with a large field of view.

Images may be electronically zoomed to magnify the image, sometimes aiding interpretation. Pinhole images will increase resolution when examining small parts such as the femoral head in children or when examining the feet and hands. There are disadvantages of pinhole imaging, including the long acquisition time needed, the limited field of view, the distortion of the image peripherally and the time to change collimators.

Planar imaging

This is the commonest type of imaging performed for bone scans and is obtained with the camera positioned as close to the patient as possible. Each image is acquired over several minutes without movement. The image obtained shows the part closest to the camera. This differs from plain X-ray; for example, the posterior view demonstrates the posterior structures, rather than the full anteroposterior thickness. The image is displayed as if the observer was the camera. For example, in a posterior view, the right side is on the observer's right, and in an anterior image the right side is on the observer's left.

SPECT imaging

The images of single photon emission computed tomography (SPECT) are acquired as the gamma camera rotates around the object. The data is then reconstructed to form three-dimensional images that can be displayed in any plane. Axial, sagittal and coronal planes are generally used, but the axis of reconstruction can be altered to relate to the anatomical structure rather than an orthogonal plane. Images are orientated in the same way as in CT and MRI.

Traditionally, filtered back-projection techniques have been used for reconstruction but newer systems using iterative reconstruction (ordered subset estimation maximisation, OSEM) reduce artefacts and noise levels. Acquisition orbits may be circular, elliptical or body contoured and the acquisition matrix is usually 128×128. Multihead cameras reduce the time necessary for SPECT acquisition.

SPECT has a definite role in many areas, aiding both detection and localisation of abnormalities. This technique plays a major role in imaging lumbar spine injuries. It must be remembered that although it improves the contrast resolution of lesions, it degrades the spatial resolution. SPECT does not replace planar imaging but is used as a helpful adjunct.

Which camera?

Although any gamma camera can be used for sports medicine imaging, a camera that allows easy rotation and versatile head tilt provides maximum ease of correct positioning. The positioning of the camera head in the closest proximity to the area of interest is absolutely essential for maximal resolution. Single head cameras are usually the most adaptable. If using a dual head camera, it is important not to use the second head to obtain the opposite lateral or oblique view, as this will not be optimally positioned close to the patient and an inferior image will be obtained.

The three-phase bone scan

Most sports medicine nuclear medicine requires three phase imaging—the flow study, the blood pool view and the delayed view. Occasionally a fourth phase or 24-hour view may be helpful.

The flow study is the set of images obtained as the radiopharmaceutical flows into the part in question. This phase will occur in the 60 seconds following injection and the authors' routine is to obtain images with 3-second frames.

The blood pool image is obtained immediately after the flow study and demonstrates relative tissue vascularity and tissue perfusion. Delay in imaging at this stage results in early bone uptake being visualised, rather than true blood pool. In many instances this image will increase the specificity of the delayed image. It may also alert the reporter and technologist to unsuspected pathology, allowing them to tailor the delayed views to achieve optimal diagnostic information. Occasionally the blood pool image may be the only abnormality in the entire study. This can be seen in paediatric imaging and in very early fractures. The blood pool image also shows the extent of the soft tissue component of the injury. For example, conditions such as tendinosis, which may have a normal or near-normal delayed image, can have a characteristic pattern on the early view, allowing an accurate diagnosis to be made. Orthogonal views should be obtained to allow better localisation of the site of increased blood pool activity.

The delayed views are performed after 2 hours and most commonly at about 3 hours post-injection to allow for maximum uptake into bone and, more importantly, clearance from extraosseous tissues.

Patient positioning is extremely important and will be addressed in detail in each chapter. In general, images should be obtained in positions which allow best visualisation without interference from overlying structures and which allow the part of interest to be as close to the camera head as possible. Traditionally, anterior, posterior and lateral images are obtained, but occasionally oblique, plantar, palmar, extra tilt or subpubic views may be necessary.

High-count images will give the best image quality. The optimal count density is always a compromise between the time a patient will tolerate immobility and the count density achievable for good quality images. Thus the count density in spinal or pelvic imaging is different from that practically achievable in hand imaging. 900K images may be obtained in spinal imaging but 300K images of the hands can sometimes exceed the time that can be tolerated by the patient. With pinhole imaging 100K images may be all that can be achieved.

Ideally, the physician should be actively involved in the decision regarding the acceptable count density on a case-to-case basis.

A fourth phase or 24-hour images may be used to see the pelvis with the bladder empty or to allow for greater clearance from extraosseous tissues. SPECT imaging usually circumvents the need for these views.

How extensively should we image?

One of the great advantages of the bone scan is that images distant from the part in question can be easily obtained without additional irradiation. The minimum extent of imaging should be at least one anatomic region above and below the part in question. For example, imaging of the feet and ankles should also include the knees and knee imaging should include the pelvis, feet and ankles.

Certain conditions can have associated injuries. For example, a fracture of the radial head or neck may be associated with a wrist fracture. Similarly, a fracture of the proximal fibular shaft may be associated with an ankle injury (a Maisonneuve fracture). The full extent of injury must be demonstrated.

Sometimes the clinician may suspect an injury at one site without realising that the symptoms have been referred from elsewhere. Situations such as knee pain referred from the hip or hip pain coming from the lumbar spine are common causes of clinical confusion. Bone scans can be extremely helpful in these cases.

Occasionally, patients referred for bone scan imaging of a particular area may be shown to have unexpected widespread skeletal abnormalities. For example, processes such as neoplasm, Paget's disease or other metabolic bone disease may be demonstrated. If indicated, a whole body study should be completed as there is no additional radiation involved.

In active people with sports injuries, more extensive imaging will demonstrate previously unknown subclinical changes. It is, however, a vexed philosophical

question whether whole-body imaging should be performed. It is not our usual practice to perform whole-body imaging because of the realities of reimbursement by government or insurance agencies unless the findings in one area could be a part of a generalised process.

Radiation dosage and radiation risks

Radiation dosimetry, radiation effects and relative risks from radiation, both from X-rays and nuclear medicine procedures, are complex technical subjects, with the details being beyond the scope of this atlas. However, in an attempt to put the subject into some perspective for the referring physicians and their patients, a brief discussion follows.

Nuclear medicine procedures use gamma rays emitted from radioactive isotopes. Gamma rays are a form of ionising radiation similar to X-rays. The activity or amount of a radioactive substance is measured in becquerels (Bq). When the radiation is absorbed in an object, the radiation absorbed dose is measured in grays (Gy). Different types of radiation have different biological effects and the equivalent dose is a quantity that takes this relative biological effect into account. This is measured in sieverts (Sv) and for ionising radiation used in medical imaging, the equivalent dose in sieverts is numerically equal to the absorbed dose in grays. Most equivalent doses used in diagnostic medical imaging are in the millisievert (mSv) or microsievert (µSv) range. The effective dose is a value calculated to take into account the relative radio-sensitivity of different organs and non-uniform dose distribution to provide an overall risk-related parameter. The non-SI units for these quantities are millicuries, rads and rems respectively (1 mCi = 37 MBq, 1 rad = 10 mGy, 1 rem = 10 Sv).

We are all exposed to radiation constantly. There is a wide range in natural background radiation, which typically averages around 2 to 3 mSv/year. Diagnostic X-rays provide approximately 10% of the average population dose and nuclear medicine about 4%. The other 86% comes from natural sources such as cosmic radiation, radiation from rocks and soils, radon and internal radiation in our bodies.

Recommended dose limits for radiation exposure to radiation workers and the general public are set by the International Commission on Radiological Protection (ICRP). For radiation workers this is 20 mSv/year and for the public 1 mSv/year averaged over 5 years.

The effective dose for a bone scan is 6.4 mSv. This is of the same order of magnitude as for lumbar spine X-rays and CT scans, more than for a chest X-ray and less than most angiography.

An alternative way of looking at the risks is to equate the theoretical radiation risk to risks of other daily activities, expressed in terms of lost life expectancy (LLE) in days:

	LLE (days)
Cigarette smoking (male) one or more packs a day	2441
15% overweight	777
Motor vehicle accident	205
Air travel (400 000 km over 40 years)	64
Passive smoking	50
Medical radiation (2 mSv/year over working life)	17
Asthma	11
Medical radiation (single exposure of 10 mSv)	**2**
Lightning strike	1
Airbag in car	−50

Radiation risk data is generally extrapolated from the known risks of exposure at higher dose levels, such as from studying the effects following the atomic bomb blasts in Japan and the Marshall Islands. Risks at lower levels are then generally extrapolated using a linear model, to obtain estimates of risk. Accurate risk assessment at low levels is difficult to obtain. There is also evidence of beneficial effects of low-level radiation, called radiation hormesis. Low levels of radiation stimulate DNA repair processes and hence the true risks of low-level radiation may be much less than those calculated.

As with any test, treatment or procedure, the potential benefit to the patient must outweigh the risks. In sports medicine this means that the information needed from a bone scan in helping to make or confirm a diagnosis, exclude other pathology and provide information and/or reassurance to the patient and doctor must outweigh the small potential risks of radiation exposure. Such radiation must then be kept as low as reasonably achievable to obtain the appropriate information.

For further technical details on nuclear medicine, the reader is referred to general texts on nuclear medicine.

Bibliography

Fogelman, I, ed., *Bone scanning in Clinical Practice*, Springer Verlag, Heidelberg, 1987

Murray, IPC, Ell, PJ, *Nuclear Medicine in Clinical Diagnosis and Treatment*, Churchill Livingstone, Edinburgh, 1998, pp. 1125–53

Rosenthal, L, Lisbona R, *Skeletal Imaging: Current Practice in Nuclear Medicine*, Appleton-Century-Crofts, Norwalk, Connecticut, 1984

2 Concepts in sports medicine imaging

3 The ankle, foot and heel

The ankle and foot are the most commonly injured areas in sport. Imaging is usually required to assess the severity of the injury, to guide management and to help estimate when the athlete may be expected to return to sport. Acute injuries are most often seen in agility sports such as basketball and football, with more chronic overuse injuries commonly originating from track and field.

Injuries involve soft tissue structures as well as bone and joints and may be difficult to diagnose on plain films, so if clinical suspicion persists following normal initial plain films, other imaging methods are employed. Bone scans play a significant role, particularly in the detection or exclusion of occult fractures.

Tips on technique

All imaging methods require attention to detail and nuclear medicine imaging of the ankle and foot is no exception. Invariably, the more care taken with technique, the greater the value of the examination. Commonly, there can be difficulty in the accurate anatomical placement of an area of increased uptake in the tarsal region when positioning is poor.

Routinely, anterior, lateral, medial and plantar views are obtained. Posterior views may be added. In all views, it is important to have the collimator as close to the object as possible (Fig. 3.1).

Anterior view

The anterior view requires the ankles to be extended as much as possible. One way to achieve this is to place the heels over the end of the bed with the patient supine. This allows for greater extension of the ankle joints in the less flexible patients.

Care should be taken to position the feet symmetrically, so that a direct comparison can be made. Being commonly injured, the lateral malleoli must always be visualised, and this is achieved by internally rotating the feet about 15 to 20 degrees, giving heel separation, preferably without inversion. To help maintain this position, the toes are held loosely together by a tourniquet to decrease the likelihood of movement. This places the talus in the true AP axis and enables the ankle joint to be viewed in the 'mortise' position. In practice, the foot is correctly positioned when the lateral border of the foot is at right angles to the bed.

Lateral and medial views

The compromise of 'skiers' views is the most common positioning for lateral and medial views. The feet are positioned one behind the other with as little obliquity as possible. Tilting of the camera is essential in obtaining adequate views, the degree of tilt varying with each patient.

In some conditions such as sesamoiditis, or subtalar pathology, a true medial or lateral view is important to obtain. In these cases, to allow precise positioning, it is best to image only the foot in question with the foot lying in direct contact with the collimator.

A 'frogleg' view is a variation to allow simultaneous acquisition of medial views. This view is useful for flow studies and blood pool images, particularly when the hind foot is the targeted area. Correct positioning requires the soles of the feet to be opposed with slight separation.

Plantar view

For plantar views, the patient is usually seated or lying on the end of the imaging table with the feet placed directly on the upturned collimator. The knees should be kept together to avoid inversion of the feet. This view is particularly useful for imaging forefoot abnormalities.

Posterior view

When obtained, the posterior view can be acquired with the patient supine and the feet extending beyond the bed. The heels are slightly separated, resting on the upturned collimator face. Plantar flexion of the feet should be avoided. This view is useful for further evaluation of ankle joint pathology.

Flow study positions

- Anterior is the preferred position for the demonstration of ankle and midfoot abnormality.
- Plantar is the position used to best demonstrate forefoot changes.
- Frogleg positioning helps demonstrate abnormality in the heel.

It is important to remember that if the patient has been on crutches prior to imaging, blood flow to the limb may be markedly reduced. In this instance it may be necessary to obtain an additional blood pool image of the pathological limb alone.

Figure 3.1 Standard views.

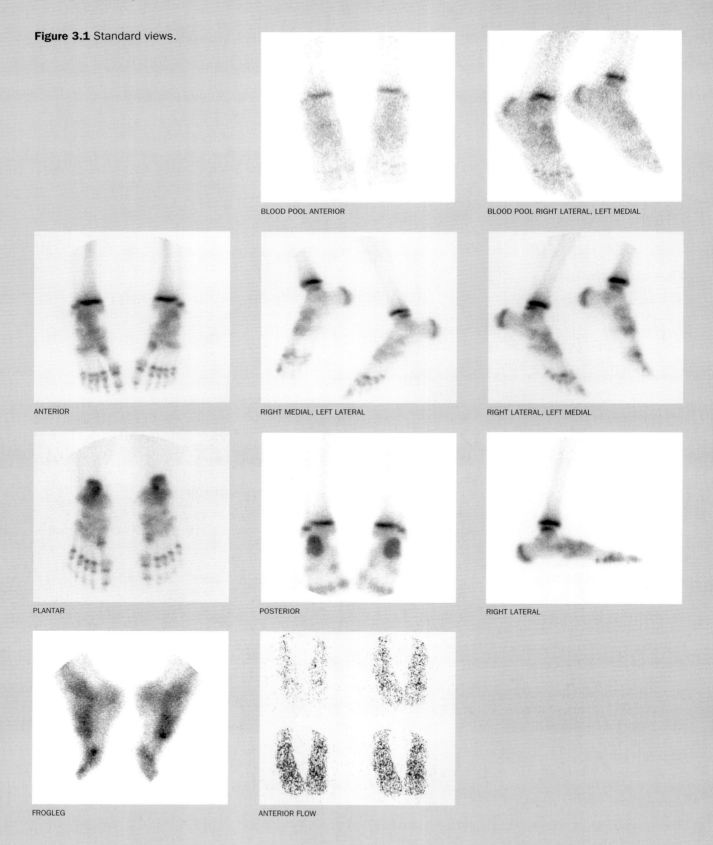

BLOOD POOL ANTERIOR

BLOOD POOL RIGHT LATERAL, LEFT MEDIAL

ANTERIOR

RIGHT MEDIAL, LEFT LATERAL

RIGHT LATERAL, LEFT MEDIAL

PLANTAR

POSTERIOR

RIGHT LATERAL

FROGLEG

ANTERIOR FLOW

Ligament injuries of the ankle and foot

Lateral ligament complex injury is the commonest injury in sport and a bone scan is not required to image the vast majority of sprains. However, delayed recovery from what appears to be a simple sprain may be due to an occult fracture. The chance of a fracture being present increases if there is a persisting effusion. In this clinical setting, a bone scan is indicated and the pattern of uptake will demonstrate the site of trauma.

A continuum of patterns is seen, ranging from incomplete ligament injuries characterised by mildly increased blood flow but normal delayed image to marked uptake on delayed images demonstrating associated bone injury. The bone injury may be at the bony attachment of the ligament or present elsewhere in the ankle joint or foot (Figs 3.2–3.4).

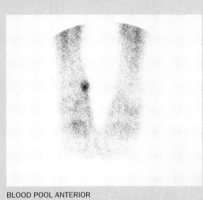

BLOOD POOL ANTERIOR

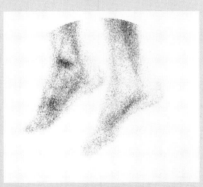

BLOOD POOL RIGHT MEDIAL, LEFT LATERAL

Figure 3.2 Soft tissue injury to the ankle. There is increased blood flow seen in the blood pool images but no focal increase in uptake in bone. There is evidence of ligament and soft tissue contusion but no bony change.

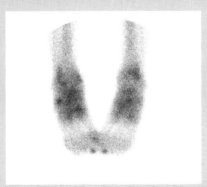

ANTERIOR

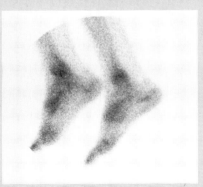

RIGHT MEDIAL, LEFT LATERAL

Figure 3.3 Ligament and malleolar injury. There is increased blood flow and increased uptake in the delayed views in the left medial malleolus, with lesser uptake in the tip of the lateral malleolus and medial and lateral edges of the talus. These changes are typical of ankle sprain with a combination of impaction- and traction-type injuries. It is frequently not possible to differentiate the mechanism of the injury on the scan. Diffuse uptake throughout the rest of the ankle joint is consistent with traumatic synovitis. Note that the medial uptake is commonly anteromedial, giving an appearance similar to anterior impingement on the medial view. Note also the mild Achilles enthesopathy.

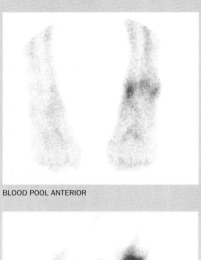

BLOOD POOL ANTERIOR

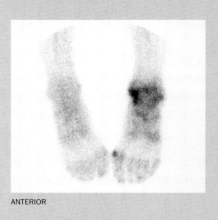

ANTERIOR

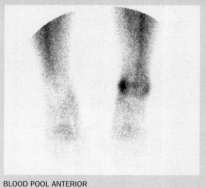

RIGHT LATERAL, LEFT MEDIAL

Figure 3.4 Traumatic synovitis, ligamentous injury and fracture at the tip of the left medial malleolus. Note that the low-grade uptake on the medial and lateral edges of the talar body, adjacent to the tips of the malleoli, may be due to traction- or impaction-type injuries. The anterior view excludes fracture in the talar dome.

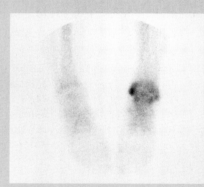

BLOOD POOL ANTERIOR

ANTERIOR

RIGHT LATERAL, LEFT MEDIAL

Ankle and foot fractures

A major role of nuclear medicine imaging is the identification of bone injury that cannot be demonstrated on plain films. This method of imaging is particularly valuable around the ankle joint and in the tarsal region, where there are curved surfaces and generally complex anatomy. Occult fractures are commonly seen around the ankle joint and are sometimes overlooked on plain films.

With increasing experience with MRI of the ankle, foot and heel in the elite athlete, a better understanding of marrow changes following both acute and chronic injury has developed. Oedema in the bone marrow may be caused by bone stress from chronic repetitive trauma or by a 'bone bruise' from a direct acute injury. These changes can be identified only by bone scan or MRI. Bone scans have the same sensitivity as MRI in demonstrating these processes and have the added advantage of being extremely cost effective. Areas of bone stress in the ankle, foot and heel in a highly trained athlete are very common and this is particularly so in the adolescent. In fact, scattered low-level areas of increased uptake in this group must be considered almost 'normal'.

All bone injury is identified on bone scan by showing an increase in uptake in the delayed images. The more severe and acute injuries usually also show an increase in the flow and blood pool phases. Low-grade injuries show a lesser degree of increase in flow, blood pool and delayed uptake.

Occult fractures of the ankle and foot (Figs 3.5–3.34)

Occult fractures are characteristically found in athletes when an ankle 'sprain' is slow to respond to treatment. These fractures often involve:

- the medial and lateral malleoli;
- the talar dome;
- the tibial plafond;
- the anterior process of the calcaneum;
- the posterior process of the talus;
- the talar body, head and neck;
- the lateral process of the talus;
- the base of the fifth metatarsal.

Figure 3.5 Small medial talar dome fracture with focal increase in blood pool activity and increase in delayed uptake localised to the medial talar dome.

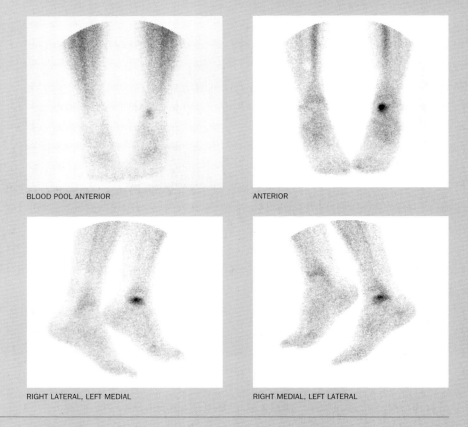

BLOOD POOL ANTERIOR

ANTERIOR

RIGHT LATERAL, LEFT MEDIAL

RIGHT MEDIAL, LEFT LATERAL

Figure 3.6 Bone bruise in the talar dome resulting from an inversion injury. This is a Stage 1 talar dome fracture. The plain film is normal and the MRI shows a geographical bone bruise, with a line of demarcation between normal and abnormal bone.

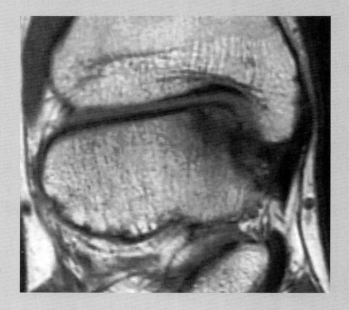

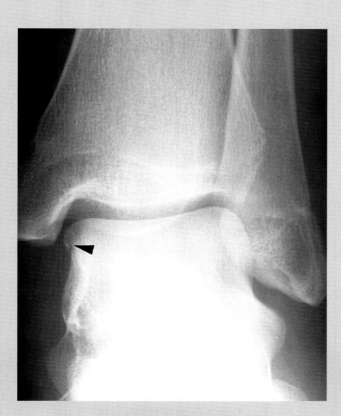

Figure 3.7 A talar dome fracture may be difficult to identify on plain films, even in retrospect, and is often overlooked.

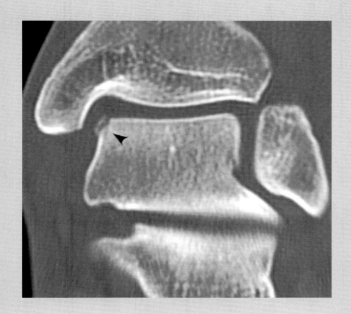

Figure 3.8 A subtle Stage 3 talar dome fracture is shown by CT.

Figure 3.9 Talar dome fracture. Note how the increase in uptake flares into the body of the talus but is most intense in the talar dome. Adjusting the image window settings in the anterior views highlights the location of the fracture in the talar dome.

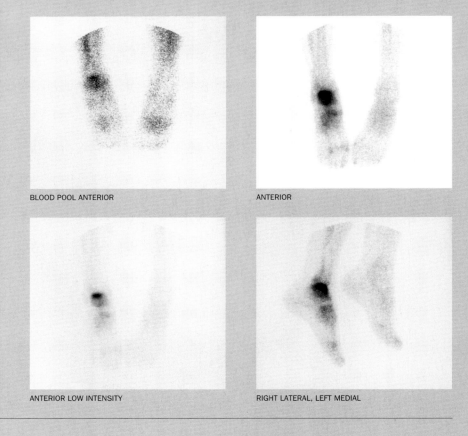

BLOOD POOL ANTERIOR

ANTERIOR

ANTERIOR LOW INTENSITY

RIGHT LATERAL, LEFT MEDIAL

Figure 3.10 Talar dome fracture. In this case the fracture line is less obvious, yet the greatest uptake is still in the dome and flares into the body of the talus.

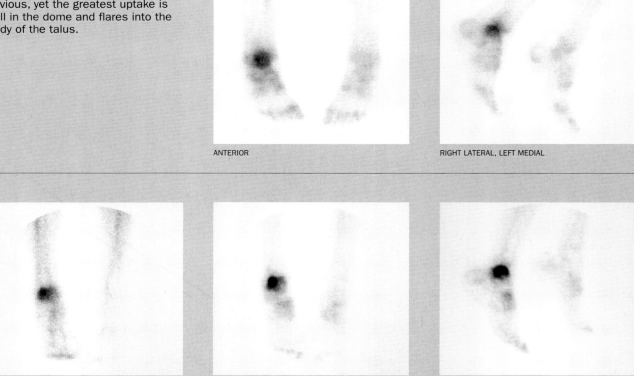

ANTERIOR

RIGHT LATERAL, LEFT MEDIAL

BLOOD POOL ANTERIOR

ANTERIOR

RIGHT LATERAL, LEFT MEDIAL

Figure 3.11 Lateral talar dome fracture.

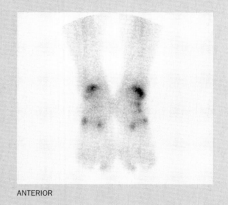

ANTERIOR

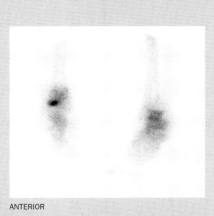

RIGHT MEDIAL, LEFT LATERAL

Figure 3.12 Bilateral talar dome fractures.

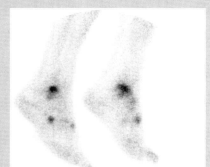

RIGHT LATERAL, LEFT MEDIAL

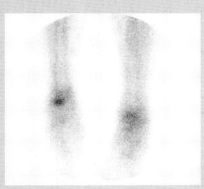

BLOOD POOL ANTERIOR

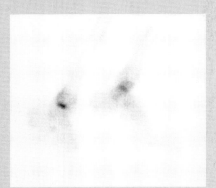

ANTERIOR

Figure 3.13 Osteochondral fracture of the distal tibia. A focus of increased blood flow and uptake of isotope localised to the articular surface of the plafond (ceiling) of the ankle joint. The blood pool and delayed uptake flare into the tibia rather than the talus.

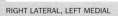

RIGHT LATERAL, LEFT MEDIAL

Figure 3.14 Osteochondral fracture of the distal tibia. Focal increase in blood flow and uptake of isotope in the anterior aspect of the distal tibia indicates fracture. Note that the activity flares into the tibia rather than the talus.

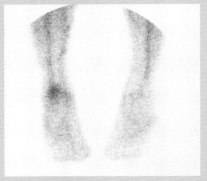

BLOOD POOL ANTERIOR

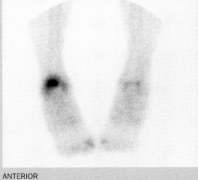

ANTERIOR

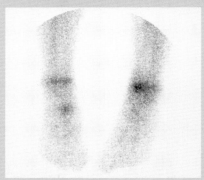

RIGHT LATERAL, LEFT MEDIAL

Figure 3.15 Epiphyseal fracture. Note the uptake in the medial part of the left distal tibial epiphysis, with only minor extension proximally into the physeal plate. This is an uncommon injury, fracture through the physeal plate being more common.

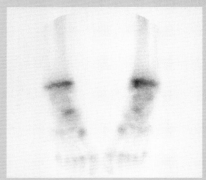

BLOOD POOL ANTERIOR

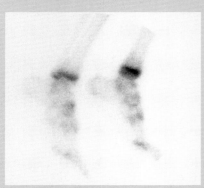

ANTERIOR

RIGHT LATERAL, LEFT MEDIAL

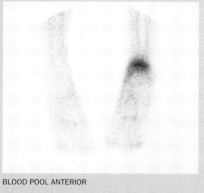

BLOOD POOL ANTERIOR

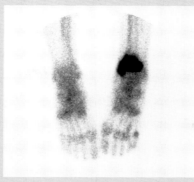

ANTERIOR

Figure 3.16 Fracture of the distal tibia close to the ankle joint but not an osteochondral fracture. There is focal increase in blood flow and uptake across the distal tibia above the ankle joint. Note how the alteration in window intensity highlights the fracture line and the flare of activity outlines the distal tibia. This was a stress fracture rather than an acute injury.

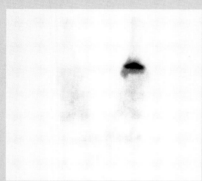

ANTERIOR LOW INTENSITY

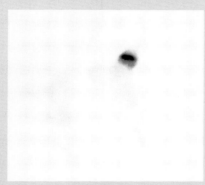

RIGHT LATERAL, LEFT MEDIAL

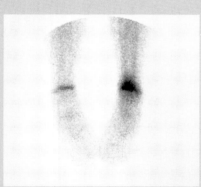

BLOOD POOL ANTERIOR

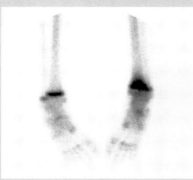

ANTERIOR

Figure 3.17 Osteomyelitis of the distal tibia. *Caution:* The appearance in this case is similar to a fracture in the distal tibia adjacent to the growth plate. This case highlights how the bone scan is non-specific and clinical correlation is always required.

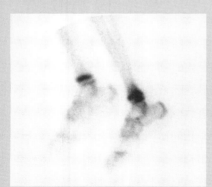

RIGHT MEDIAL, LEFT LATERAL

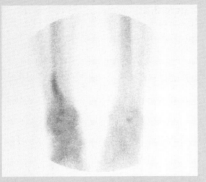

ANTERIOR

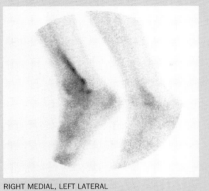

RIGHT MEDIAL, LEFT LATERAL

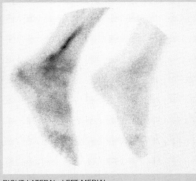

RIGHT LATERAL, LEFT MEDIAL

Figure 3.18 Vertical (spiral) fracture of the distal tibia extending to the ankle joint.

Figure 3.19 Bone stress involving the anterior process of the calcaneum. High signal in the anterior process indicates bone stress due to repetitive traction by the bifurcate ligament.
This patient is an Olympic track-and-field athlete and, at this level of sport, areas of high signal are commonly seen scattered through the bones of the feet and are more often than not asymptomatic.

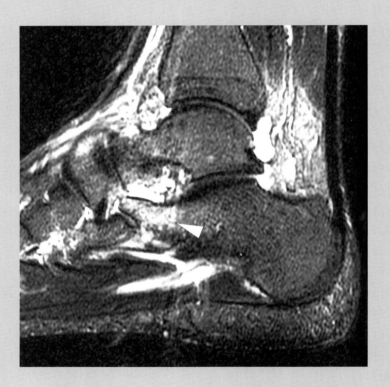

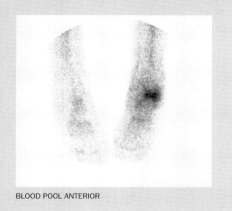

BLOOD POOL ANTERIOR

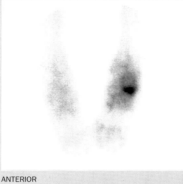

ANTERIOR

Figure 3.20 Extensive fracture of the anterior process of the left calcaneum. Note the abrupt cut-off with activity flaring from the calcaneocuboid joint back into the calcaneum and the involvement of the whole of the anterior process.

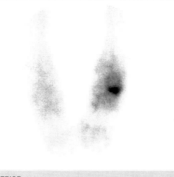

RIGHT MEDIAL, LEFT LATERAL

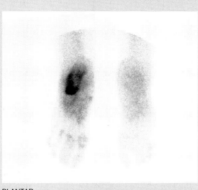

PLANTAR

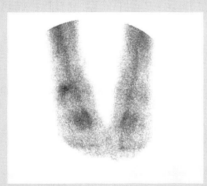

BLOOD POOL ANTERIOR

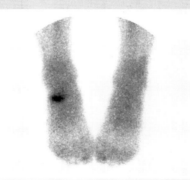

ANTERIOR

Figure 3.21 Less extensive fracture of the anterior process of the right calcaneum. In this case the appearance is more typical, being confined to the dorsal edge of the anterior process. With good localisation, the diagnosis can still be made despite poor bone uptake.

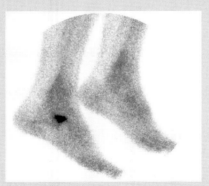

RIGHT LATERAL, LEFT MEDIAL

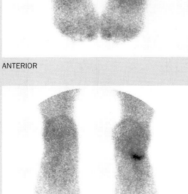

PLANTAR

Figure 3.22 A fracture of the anterior process of the calcaneum is known as the 'missed' fracture due to its reputation of avoiding detection. This fracture is best seen on the oblique view of the foot.

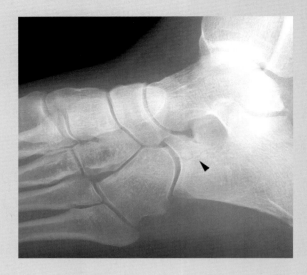

Figure 3.23 Low-grade fracture of the anterior process of the left calcaneum. There was marked reduction in blood flow to the left leg due to absent weightbearing on crutches. This is the cause of the reduced uptake in the left leg on the delayed anterior image. Imaging the symptomatic left leg separately can be a helpful technique to obtain adequate count density and provide a diagnostic quality image.

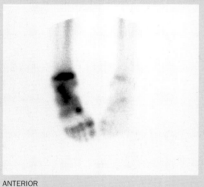

ANTERIOR

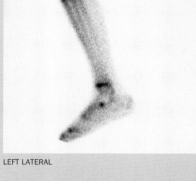

LEFT LATERAL

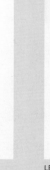

PLANTAR

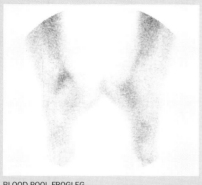

BLOOD POOL FROGLEG

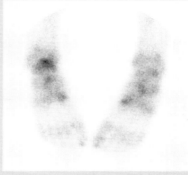

ANTERIOR

Figure 3.24 Fracture of the posterior process of the talus. Focal increase in blood flow and a focus of uptake in the posterior process of the talus with flaring into the body of the talus. Note that the lateral views are helpful in localising the exact site of the fracture and excluding a talar dome fracture.

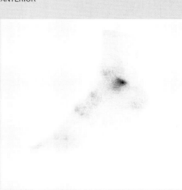

RIGHT LATERAL, LEFT MEDIAL

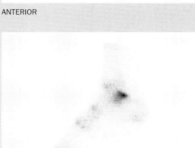

RIGHT MEDIAL

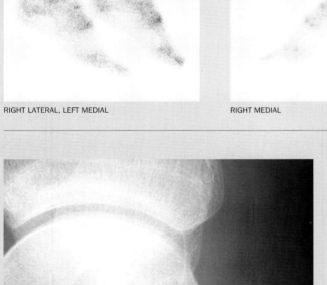

Figure 3.25 Forced plantar flexion of the ankle may result in a fracture of the posterior process of the talus. This fracture is often difficult to differentiate from an os trigonum.

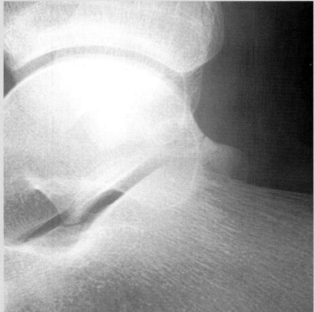

Figure 3.26 Fracture in the body of the talus. Increased blood flow and uptake of isotope in the talus in an 11-year-old patient. In the anterior projection the fracture could be mistaken for a talar dome fracture but, in the lateral view, the fracture is shown to be in the posterior talar body.

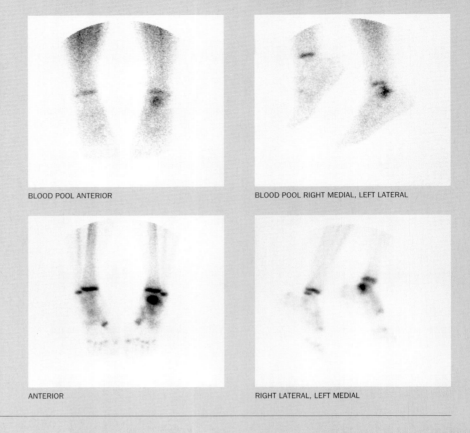

BLOOD POOL ANTERIOR

BLOOD POOL RIGHT MEDIAL, LEFT LATERAL

ANTERIOR

RIGHT LATERAL, LEFT MEDIAL

Figure 3.27 Fracture in the anterior body of the talus.

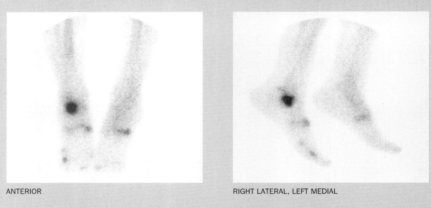

ANTERIOR

RIGHT LATERAL, LEFT MEDIAL

Figure 3.28 Fracture of the lateral process of the talus. Note also the fracture in the base of the right third metatarsal.

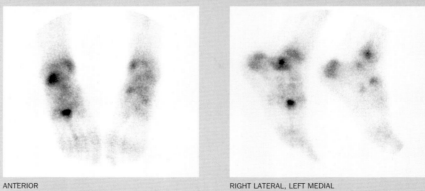

ANTERIOR

RIGHT LATERAL, LEFT MEDIAL

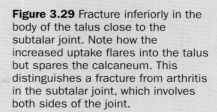

Figure 3.29 Fracture inferiorly in the body of the talus close to the subtalar joint. Note how the increased uptake flares into the talus but spares the calcaneum. This distinguishes a fracture from arthritis in the subtalar joint, which involves both sides of the joint.

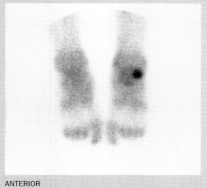

ANTERIOR

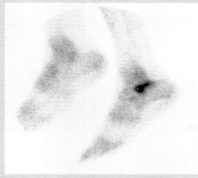

RIGHT MEDIAL, LEFT LATERAL

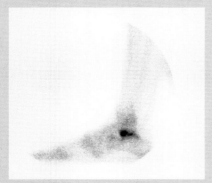

LEFT LATERAL

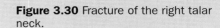

Figure 3.30 Fracture of the right talar neck.

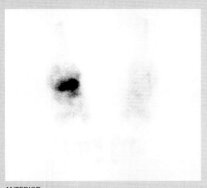

ANTERIOR

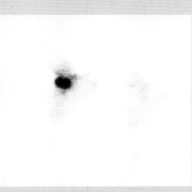

RIGHT MEDIAL, LEFT LATERAL

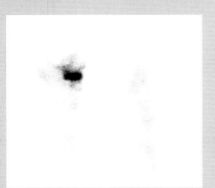

RIGHT LATERAL, LEFT MEDIAL

Figure 3.31 Bone stress is demonstrated across the neck of the talus.

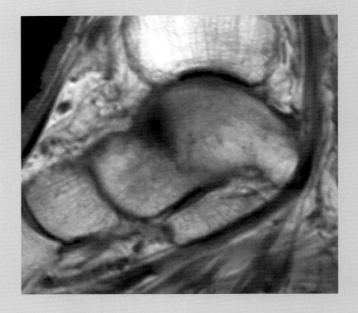

Figure 3.32 Fracture of the head and neck of the left talus. Note the abrupt cut-off at the talonavicular joint with activity flaring proximally into the talus.

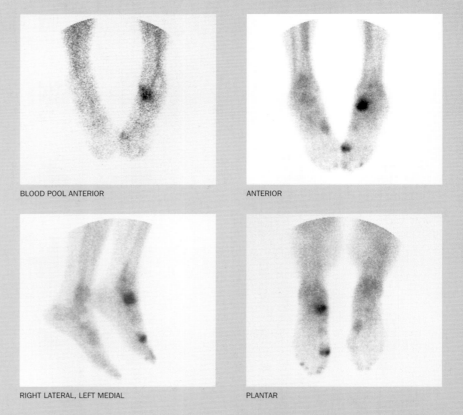

BLOOD POOL ANTERIOR

ANTERIOR

RIGHT LATERAL, LEFT MEDIAL

PLANTAR

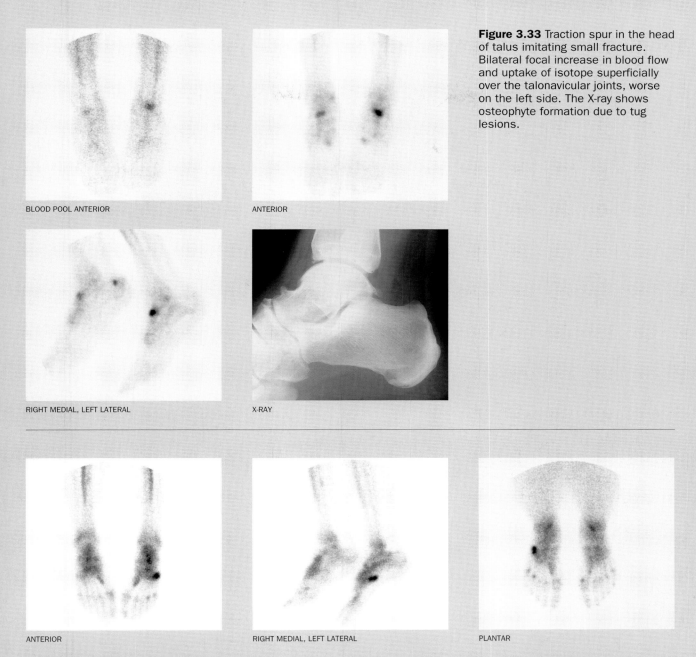

BLOOD POOL ANTERIOR

ANTERIOR

Figure 3.33 Traction spur in the head of talus imitating small fracture. Bilateral focal increase in blood flow and uptake of isotope superficially over the talonavicular joints, worse on the left side. The X-ray shows osteophyte formation due to tug lesions.

RIGHT MEDIAL, LEFT LATERAL

X-RAY

ANTERIOR

RIGHT MEDIAL, LEFT LATERAL

PLANTAR

Figure 3.34 Fracture of the base of the left fifth metatarsal. The uptake is too intense for an enthesopathy of the peroneus brevis insertion.

In the foot, acute occult fractures occur usually as a result of plantar flexion of the midfoot or midfoot twisting injury and are seen at:

· the lateral aspect of the calcaneocuboid articulation;
· the tarsometatarsal joints (particularly the second involving the Lisfranc ligament) (see below);
· the navicular tuberosity due to disruption of the os tibiale externum either by an acute or chronic injury (Fig. 3.35);
· the sesamoids due to direct trauma to this area (Fig. 3.36).

Figure 3.35 Fracture of the navicular tuberosity. This is usually an avulsion fracture at the insertion of the tibialis posterior tendon. Note there is a spectrum of activity from milder uptake in enthesopathies to greater uptake in fractures. The intensity of the localised blood pool activity and delayed bone uptake is a good guide to the degree of bony injury (fracture).

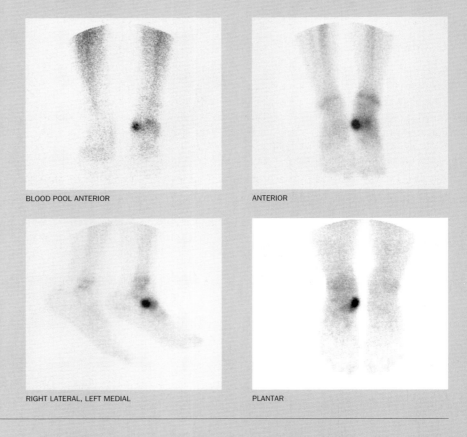

BLOOD POOL ANTERIOR   ANTERIOR

RIGHT LATERAL, LEFT MEDIAL   PLANTAR

Figure 3.36 A fracture of the medial sesamoid has resulted from direct trauma.

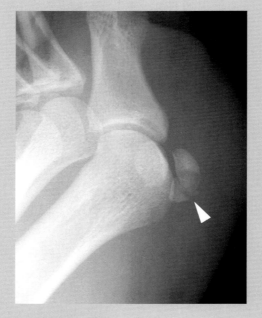

Bone stress and stress fractures of the ankle and foot

Metatarsal bone stress (Figs 3.37–3.46)

The neck of the third metatarsal is the commonest site of bone stress/stress fracture. All metatarsals can undergo stress and this process may progress to stress fracture. Foot biomechanics and variations in foot structure may contribute to the process and determine the site of stress. For example, fractures of the base of the second metatarsal occur in ballerinas with a short first metatarsal (Morton's foot). With this anomaly, when the ballerina is dancing *en pointe*, the weightbearing occurs along the second ray instead of the first and, of course, the second metatarsal is mechanically inferior. Stress fractures also involve the fifth metatarsal in the position of the Jones fracture (proximal diaphysis).

Bone scans can be helpful when plain film changes are absent or equivocal. Typically with bone stress, there is a focus of increased blood flow and increased uptake of isotope in the delayed images. This uptake usually extends along the shaft of the bone due to associated hyperaemia. This can help distinguish bone stress from either tarsometatarsal or metatarsophalangeal arthritis. Another distinguishing feature of bone stress is that it will involve only one side of a joint.

In younger patients, be aware of the persistence of physeal uptake, particularly at the base of the first metatarsal. This can persist up to the age of 17 or 18 years and asymmetrical closure of the epiphyses can also be confusing.

Figure 3.37 Right second metatarsal fracture in the midshaft.

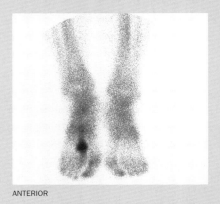 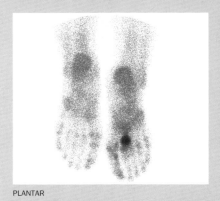

ANTERIOR   PLANTAR

Figure 3.38 Bone stress without fracture line in a marathon runner. There is increased signal in the medulla of the first metatarsal, typical of bone stress. No fracture line can be seen and the changes are indicative of trabecular level injury.

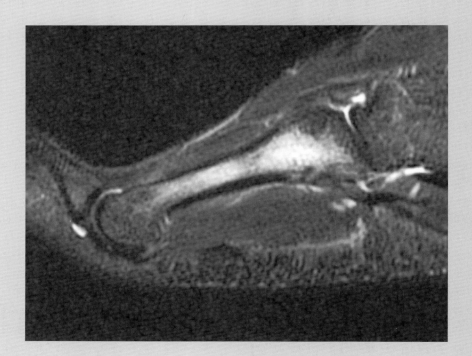

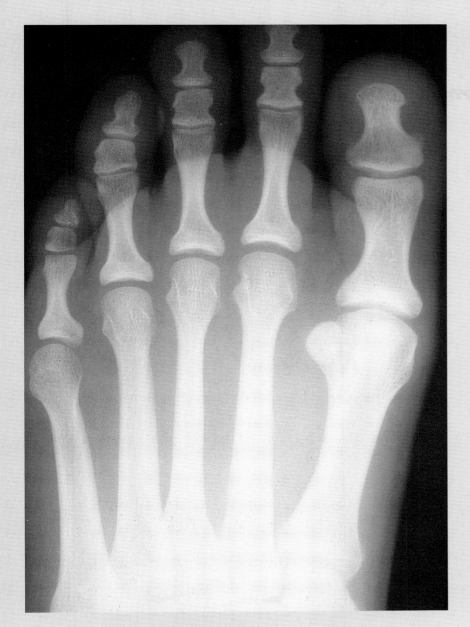

Figure 3.39 An X-ray of Morton's foot showing a short first metatarsal. When this anomaly occurs in a ballerina, problems can develop at the second tarsometatarsal joint. There can be development of either synovitis or bone stress at the base of the second metatarsal.

Figure 3.40 A young ballet dancer with a fracture in the base of the right second metatarsal. An old fracture in the left second metatarsal is also present. Note that the flaring of activity down the shaft helps distinguish a fracture from tarsometatarsal joint arthritis. If the flaring is not present it may not be possible to distinguish the two conditions on bone scan. Flaring into the shaft may also help distinguish fractures in the metatarsal head from metatarsophalangeal arthritis.

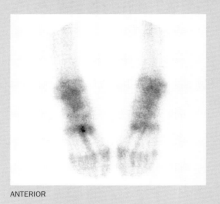
ANTERIOR

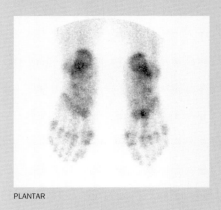
PLANTAR

Figure 3.41 Fracture of the left third metatarsal shaft distally.

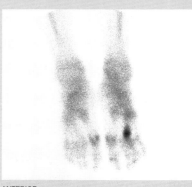
ANTERIOR

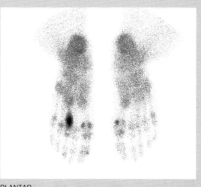
PLANTAR

Figure 3.42 A stress fracture of the third metatarsal shows a marked periosteal reaction.

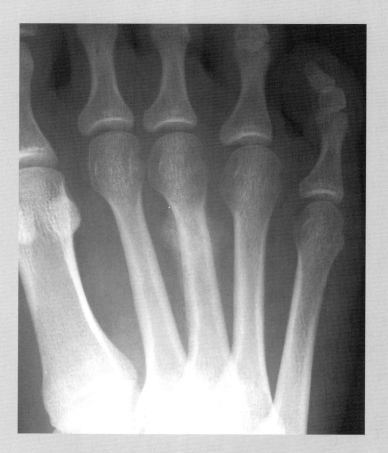

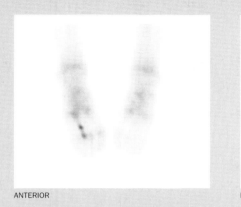 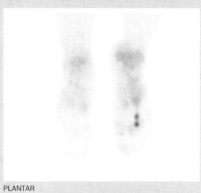

ANTERIOR

PLANTAR

Figure 3.43 Fractures in the midshaft and head of the right third metatarsal bone. This is a rare occurrence.

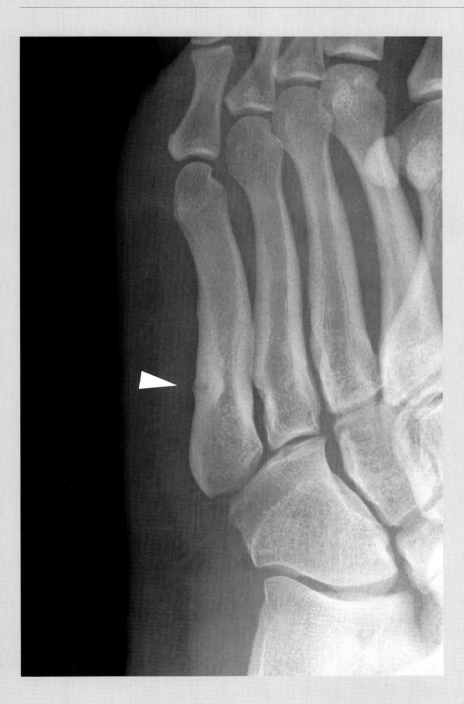

Figure 3.44 A stress fracture in the proximal diaphysis of the fifth metatarsal is prone to delayed union.

Figure 3.45 Right second metatarsal head fracture through the growth plate in a child. Both the blood pool and delayed activity are confined to the growth plate on one side of the joint only. It is important to distinguish this from osteochondritis of the second metatarsal head (Freiberg's disease), where the uptake will be in the epiphysis (distal to the physis) in the revascularising phase.

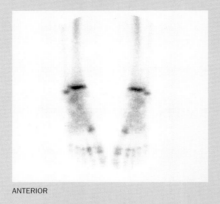
ANTERIOR

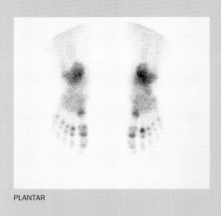
PLANTAR

Figure 3.46 Fracture in the right second toe proximal phalanx adjacent to the proximal interphalangeal joint, with activity flaring along the shaft.

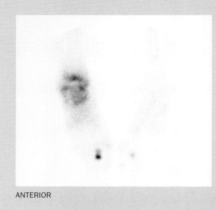
ANTERIOR

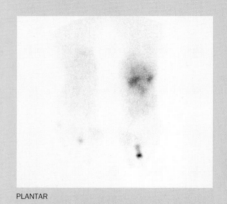
PLANTAR

Osteochondritis (Fig. 3.47)

Most commonly, this condition involves the epiphysis of the head of the second metatarsal and develops just before fusion. Other metatarsals can be involved and the site of the change presumably depends on local overloading due to biomechanics. This is an avascular process and may initially show decreased perfusion and uptake. In the stages of fragmentation, compression and healing with remodelling, the changes are indistinguishable from a fracture.

Figure 3.47 Repetitive stress on bone can produce avascular change and manifest as 'osteochondritis'. The changes shown progress through sclerosis, fragmentation and compression as the process heals.

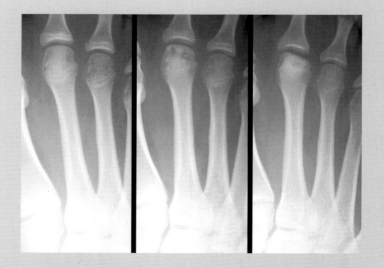

Tarsal bone stress (Figs 3.48–3.56)

Stress fractures of the navicular are surprisingly common amongst elite track-and-field athletes. The fracture is commonly bilateral and is quite often asymptomatic on one side.

Stress fractures have been described in every tarsal bone with the more common sites including the body, lateral process and neck of the talus, anterior process and tuberosity of the calcaneum, cuboid and cuneiform bones.

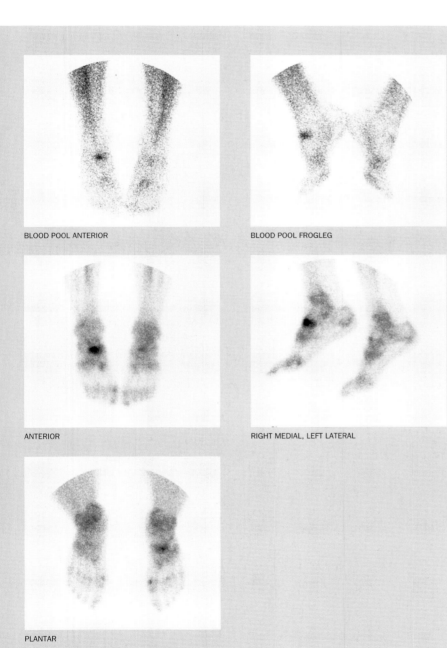

BLOOD POOL ANTERIOR

BLOOD POOL FROGLEG

ANTERIOR

RIGHT MEDIAL, LEFT LATERAL

PLANTAR

Figure 3.48 Low-grade navicular stress fracture with increased blood flow and delayed uptake, maximal at the dorsal edge of the right navicular bone.

Figure 3.49 Stress fracture. Bone stress has progressed to a detectable fracture in the left navicular.

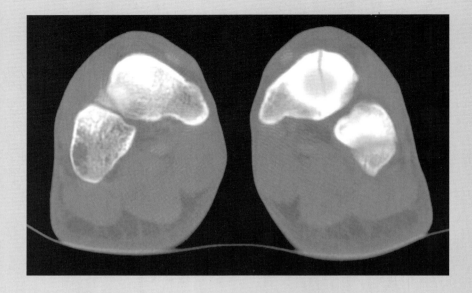

Figure 3.50 Severe navicular stress fracture with intense uptake throughout the entire navicular bone. Adjusting the window aids in localising the site of the prime pathology.

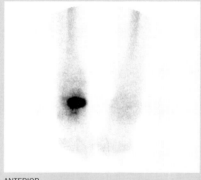

ANTERIOR

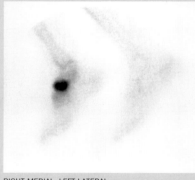

RIGHT MEDIAL, LEFT LATERAL

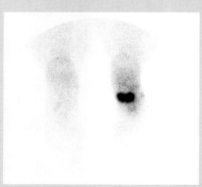

PLANTAR

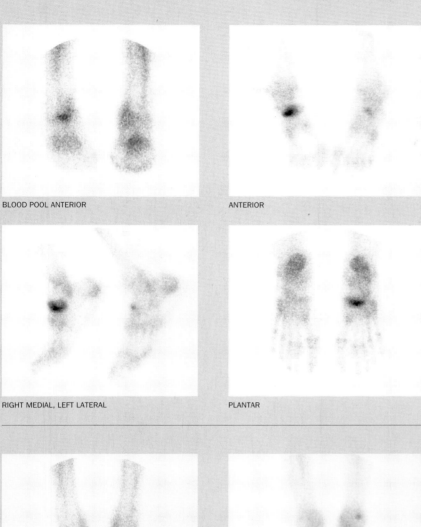

BLOOD POOL ANTERIOR

ANTERIOR

RIGHT MEDIAL, LEFT LATERAL

PLANTAR

Figure 3.51 Fracture in the right navicular distally. Note that the line of most intense activity is at the navicular-cuneiform joint, with activity flaring proximally into the navicular bone. This distinguishes fracture from arthritis, which involves both sides of the joint.

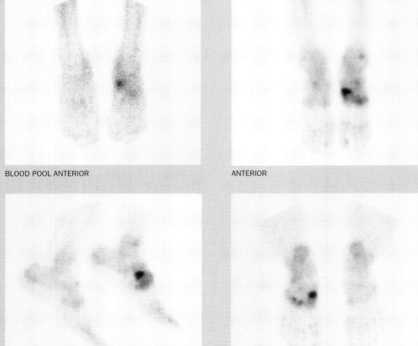

BLOOD POOL ANTERIOR

ANTERIOR

RIGHT LATERAL, LEFT MEDIAL

PLANTAR

Figure 3.52 Left medial (first) cuneiform fracture with a focal increase in vascularity and delayed uptake in the medial cuneiform. Mild uptake in the left third and fourth tarsometatarsal joints indicates associated traumatic synovitis.

Figure 3.53 Mid (second) cuneiform fracture.

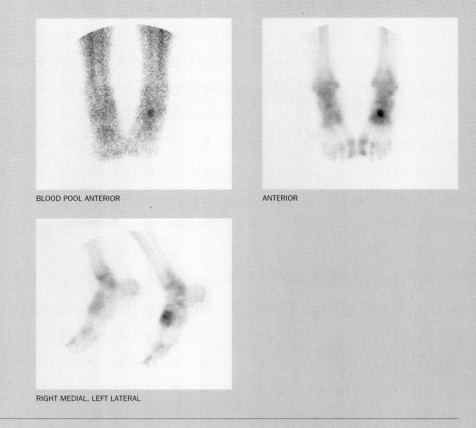

BLOOD POOL ANTERIOR

ANTERIOR

RIGHT MEDIAL, LEFT LATERAL

Figure 3.54 Lateral (third) cuneiform fracture. The plantar delayed image shows uptake flaring from the lateral inter-cuneiform joint into the lateral (third) cuneiform.

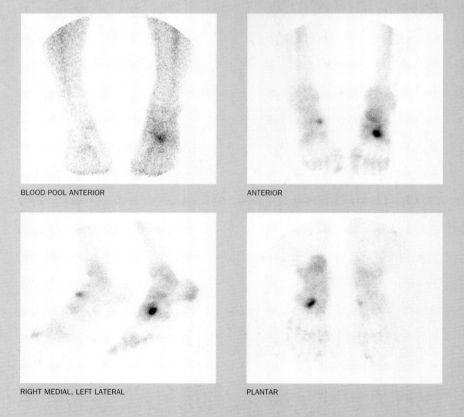

BLOOD POOL ANTERIOR

ANTERIOR

RIGHT MEDIAL, LEFT LATERAL

PLANTAR

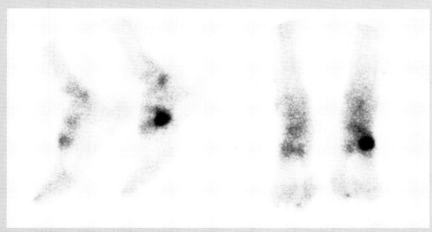

Figure 3.55 Stress fracture of the left cuboid is shown on bone scan. The CT demonstrates sclerosis at the site of bone stress.

RIGHT MEDIAL, LEFT LATERAL   ANTERIOR

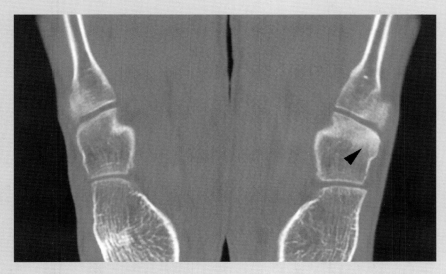

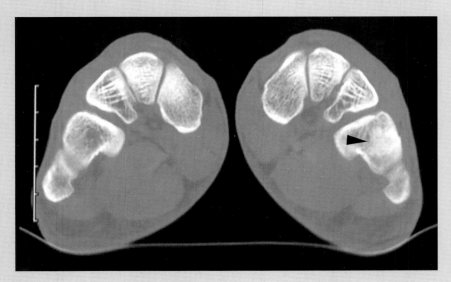

Figure 3.56 Right cuboid fracture, localised to the tuberosity.

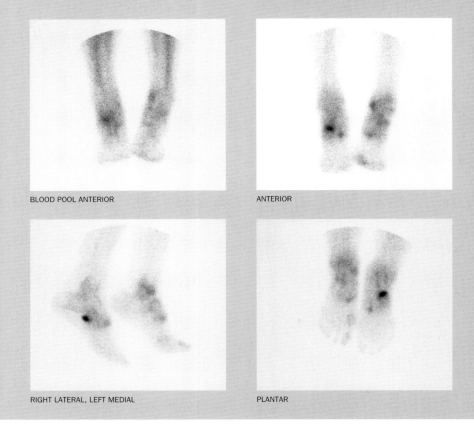

BLOOD POOL ANTERIOR

ANTERIOR

RIGHT LATERAL, LEFT MEDIAL

PLANTAR

Tendinosis and enthesopathies (Figs 3.57–3.64)

Tendinosis of the tibialis posterior and flexor hallucis longus tendons can present as ankle pain and may be unsuspected until the bone scan is performed. 'Frogleg' blood pool images can show the characteristic increase in blood flow in a linear pattern along the anatomical course of the tendon. Delayed images may be normal or, occasionally with tibialis posterior tendinosis, show a small focal increase in uptake at the tip of the medial malleolus due to hyperaemia in this region. This should not be confused with a focal bony lesion. (The characteristic early view should prevent any confusion.) There may also be increased uptake at the navicular tuberosity due to insertional enthesopathy. Enthesopathies may occur without accompanying tendinosis.

Peroneus longus tendinosis has a similar appearance on a flow study and early views. This is usually associated with a small focus of uptake laterally in the cuboid bone or in the lateral malleolus due to hyperaemia as the tendon passes adjacent to the bone.

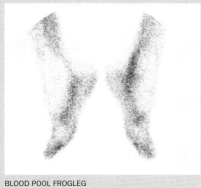

BLOOD POOL FROGLEG

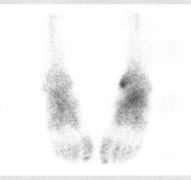

ANTERIOR

Figure 3.57 Tibialis posterior tendinosis. The blood pool images demonstrate increased vascularity along the line of the tendon. The delayed views demonstrate uptake superficially in the posterior portion of the medial malleolus, secondary to the adjacent soft tissue inflammation.

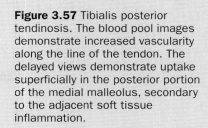

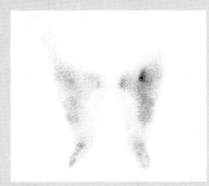

FROGLEG

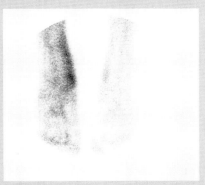

BLOOD POOL ANTERIOR

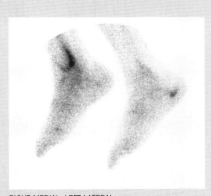

RIGHT MEDIAL, LEFT LATERAL

Figure 3.58 Severe tibialis posterior tendinosis with more extensive bony reaction extending proximally from the medial malleolus. The coexistent left plantar fasciitis may be a secondary phenomenon to altered gait.

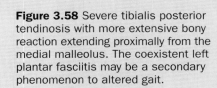

ANTERIOR

Figure 3.59 Tibialis posterior tendinosis, which extends to involve the insertion site at the navicular tuberosity (enthesopathy).

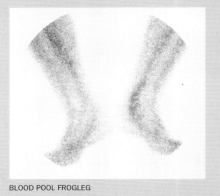
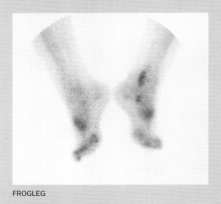

BLOOD POOL FROGLEG

FROGLEG

Figure 3.60 Bilateral navicular tuberosity enthesopathy. Traction on the fibrous junction of an accessory navicular bone with the navicular body has the same appearance and is only distinguished on X-ray. In this case the blood pool image is normal.

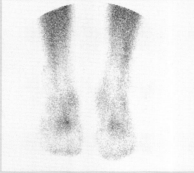
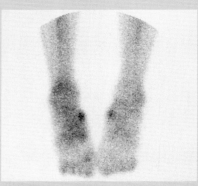

BLOOD POOL ANTERIOR

ANTERIOR

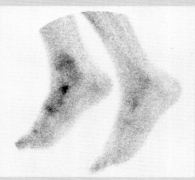
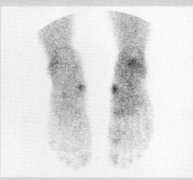

RIGHT MEDIAL, LEFT LATERAL

PLANTAR

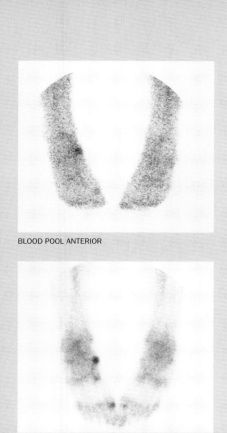

BLOOD POOL ANTERIOR

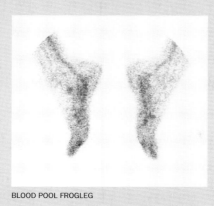

BLOOD POOL FROGLEG

Figure 3.61 Right navicular tuberosity enthesopathy showing greater vascularity and more intense uptake on the delayed images.

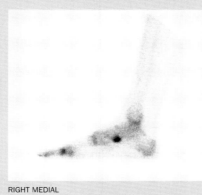

ANTERIOR

RIGHT MEDIAL

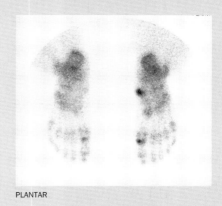

PLANTAR

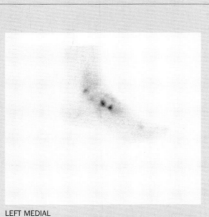

ANTERIOR

LEFT MEDIAL

Figure 3.62 Left tibialis posterior enthesopathy with uptake at both the navicular tuberosity and medial cuneiform insertion sites.

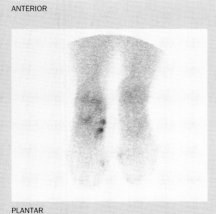

PLANTAR

Figure 3.63 Right peroneus longus tendinosis. The blood pool images show increased vascularity in the line of the peroneus longus tendon in its course in the lateral foot. The delayed images show only a mild increase in uptake in the region of the cuboid tuberosity secondary to the adjacent soft tissue hyperaemia.

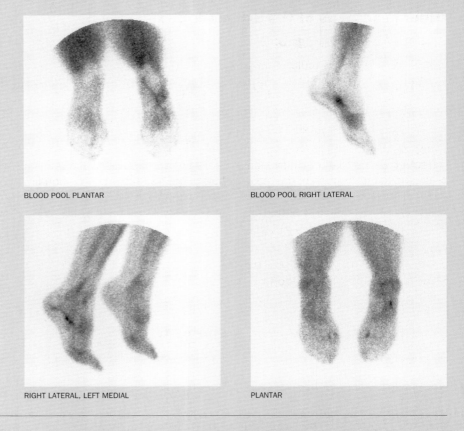

BLOOD POOL PLANTAR

BLOOD POOL RIGHT LATERAL

RIGHT LATERAL, LEFT MEDIAL

PLANTAR

Figure 3.64 Left peroneus longus tendinosis. There is linear vascularity at the lateral edge of the ankle extending around the cuboid. Greater uptake on the delayed images over the cuboid tuberosity indicates bony reaction in the cuboid bone or adjacent os peroneum.

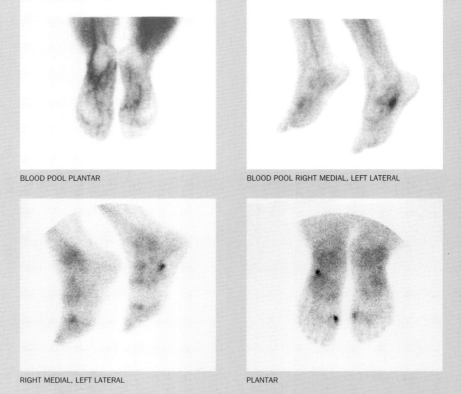

BLOOD POOL PLANTAR

BLOOD POOL RIGHT MEDIAL, LEFT LATERAL

ANTERIOR

RIGHT MEDIAL, LEFT LATERAL

PLANTAR

Other conditions of the ankle and foot

Avascular necrosis (Figs 3.65 and 3.66)

Not uncommonly, avascular changes are seen in the foot and ankle. An avascular process produces both sesamoiditis and osteochondritis. Similarly, areas of osteochondritis dissecans are seen particularly in ballet dancers and these areas are presumably the result of repetitive stress producing an avascular change.

Avascular necrosis can also involve the talus and takes two forms. Following a fracture of the talar neck, avascular changes may develop in the body of talus due to interruption of the blood supply at the fracture site. Additionally, avascular areas can develop in the subchondral bone of the talar dome. Subchondral cysts that are seen beneath chondral injury appear to develop in avascular areas of bone. A type 1 talar dome fracture may also become avascular and fragment.

In the early stages of an avascular process, uptake may be reduced or absent. With revascularisation, increased uptake in the area will become increasingly obvious.

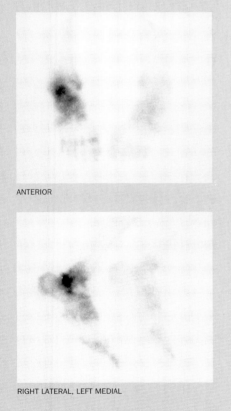

ANTERIOR

RIGHT MEDIAL, LEFT LATERAL

RIGHT LATERAL, LEFT MEDIAL

Figure 3.65 Comminuted fracture in the body of the talus with avascular necrosis of the medial dome, neck and head of the talus.

Figure 3.66 Fracture in the body of the talus with avascular necrosis anterolaterally in the talar dome.

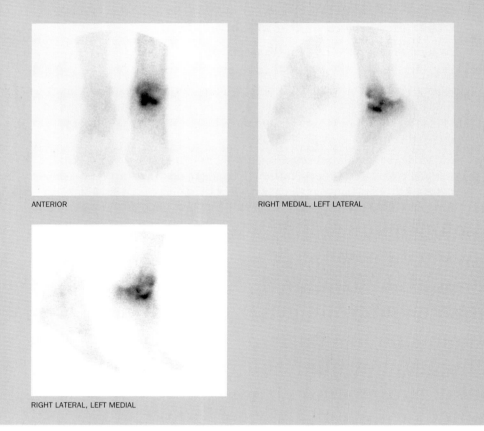

ANTERIOR

RIGHT MEDIAL, LEFT LATERAL

RIGHT LATERAL, LEFT MEDIAL

Injury to the tibiofibular syndesmosis (Figs 3.67–3.72)

This injury is often extremely difficult to recognise on plain films, and if left undiagnosed can be the cause of severe ongoing disability and early degenerative change in the ankle joint.

The mechanism of injury, with forced dorsiflexion of the ankle and/or lateral rotation of the foot, produces considerable soft tissue injury. In the flow study there is an increase in blood flow in soft tissue around the ankle joint due to rupture of ligaments and joint capsule, and a characteristic appearance of a torn interosseous ligament may be seen. The delayed images will show increased uptake in the syndesmosis with periosteal increased uptake above the syndesmosis, along the tibial shaft. There may also be injury to the posterior lip of the distal tibia. Injury to the deltoid ligament or medial malleolus fracture is usually associated.

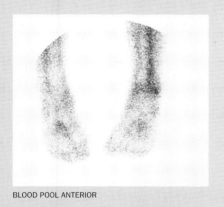
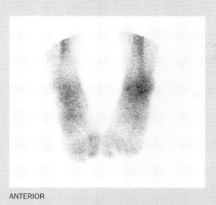
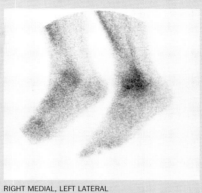

BLOOD POOL ANTERIOR   ANTERIOR   RIGHT MEDIAL, LEFT LATERAL

Figure 3.67 Disruption of the tibiofibular syndesmosis and tear of the interosseous membrane. The blood pool images show increased vascularity in the left ankle joint and a vertical linear increase in blood pool activity above the ankle joint, lateral to the tibia. In this case there is no osseous injury in the ankle joint but there is traumatic synovitis.

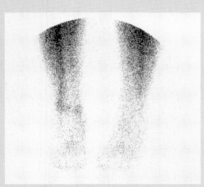
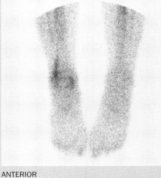

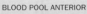
BLOOD POOL ANTERIOR   ANTERIOR

Figure 3.68 Interosseous membrane injury. Mild increase in blood pool activity, but with a greater increase in periosteal activity at the interosseous membrane attachment on the right tibia on the delayed views.

Figure 3.69 Calcification is seen in the interosseous ligament (X-ray).

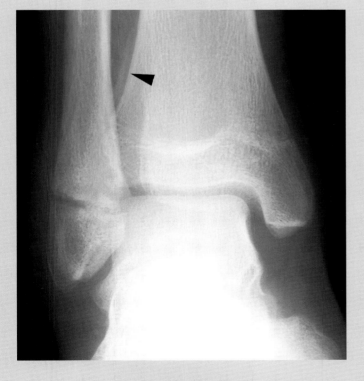

Figure 3.70 Interosseous membrane injury with posterior malleolar fracture. The linear increase in blood pool activity indicates tear of the right interosseous membrane. The delayed images show periosteal increase in uptake in the lateral side of the tibia. There is a low-grade fracture in the posterior malleolus of the distal tibia. This occurs commonly with this injury.

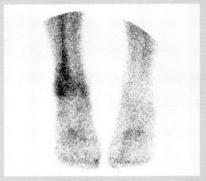
BLOOD POOL ANTERIOR

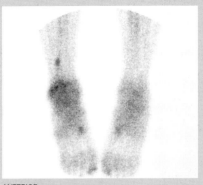
ANTERIOR

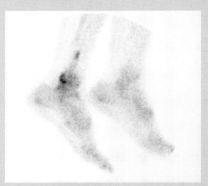
RIGHT LATERAL, LEFT MEDIAL

Figure 3.71 The presence of an isolated fracture of the posterior lip of the distal tibia may be indicative of a syndesmosis injury, representing avulsion by the posterior tibiofibular ligament.

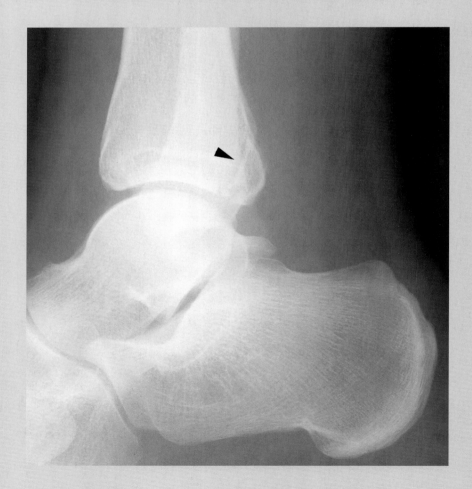

THE ANKLE, FOOT AND HEEL

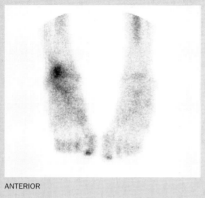

ANTERIOR

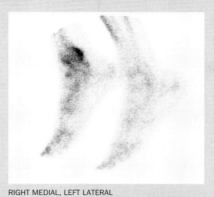

RIGHT MEDIAL, LEFT LATERAL

Figure 3.72 A more severe posterior malleolar fracture with only minor periosteal uptake at the inter-osseous membrane attachment.

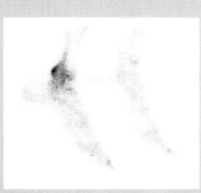

RIGHT LATERAL, LEFT MEDIAL

Maisonneuve fracture (Figs 3.73–3.75)

This is a spiral fracture of the proximal fibula associated with a syndesmosis injury. This fracture results from a rotational torque through the fibula as a result of the lateral rotation of the foot and rupturing of the distal tibiofibular ligaments. The same force can sometimes tear the interosseous ligament up to the level of the fibular fracture. Following this type of injury, the necessity to image beyond the ankle joint is highlighted. The fibular fracture may be undetected unless an extensive regional image is obtained. Injury to the interosseous ligament should also be imaged throughout its length as the extent of the injury has important prognostic implications.

Figure 3.73 Maisonneuve fracture. Spiral fracture in the proximal fibula and fracture in the tibial plafond. There is reduced bone uptake in the left leg due to absent weightbearing on crutches. The spiral fracture in the proximal fibula was clinically unsuspected because the ankle injury was too painful for weightbearing.

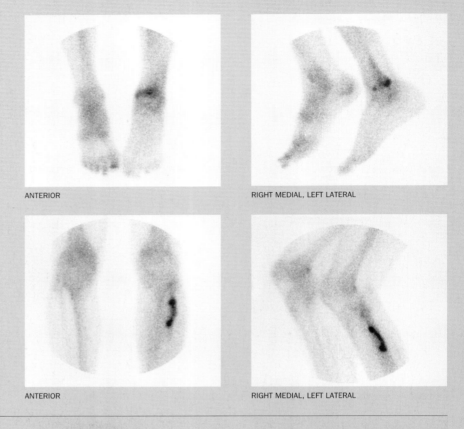

ANTERIOR

RIGHT MEDIAL, LEFT LATERAL

ANTERIOR

RIGHT MEDIAL, LEFT LATERAL

Figure 3.74 (right and opposite page) Progressive external rotation of the foot will produce injury in a sequential fashion and may progress to producing a spiral fracture of the fibular shaft (Maisonneuve fracture).

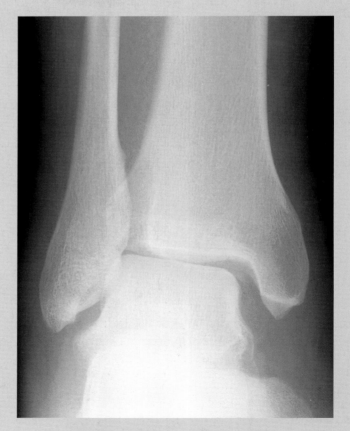

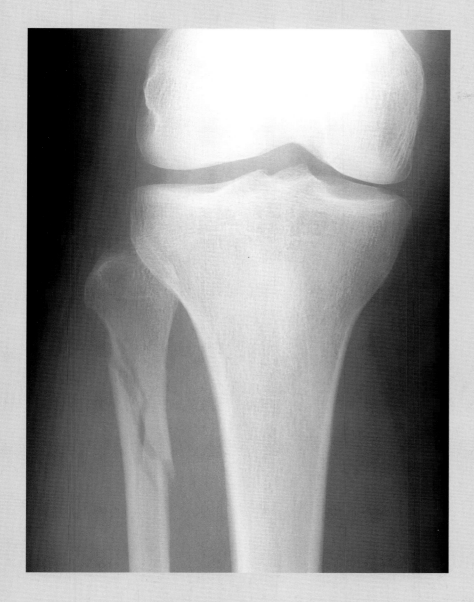

Figure 3.75 Talar fracture with fracture in the proximal fibular head. Trauma to the lateral compartment of the right knee is noted.

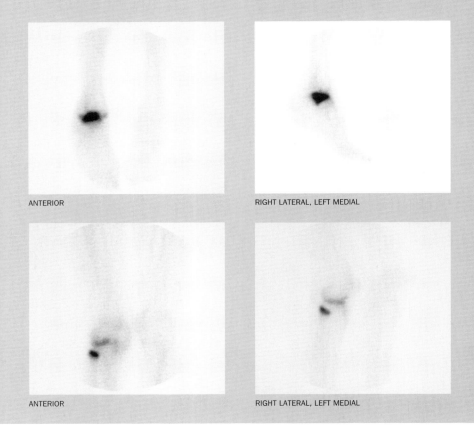

ANTERIOR

RIGHT LATERAL, LEFT MEDIAL

ANTERIOR

RIGHT LATERAL, LEFT MEDIAL

Impingement syndromes

Ankle impingement occurs most commonly on the anterior and posterior aspects of the joint. Lateral and medial impingement are also occasionally encountered.

Impingement is a clinical diagnosis, with pain and disability occurring with certain ankle movements and positions. Both bony and soft tissue structures contribute to impingement, and post-traumatic changes in these tissues can be demonstrated on bone scan. Plain films can sometimes demonstrate bony abutment using impingement (functional) views, but the soft tissue contribution to the process cannot be assessed.

Anterior impingement syndrome (Figs 3.76 and 3.77)

In athletes, particularly footballers, bony spurs can develop at the anterior aspect of the distal tibia and also on the dorsal aspect of the neck of the talus. These spurs develop as 'tug' lesions at the anterior capsular attachments and impingement may occur with dorsiflexion of the ankle. Synovitis may also contribute to this impingement.

The bone scan may show a focus or foci of increased uptake of isotope at the joint margins.

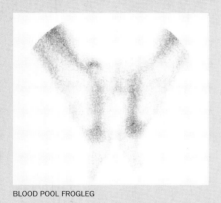

BLOOD POOL FROGLEG

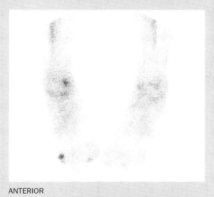

ANTERIOR

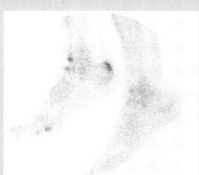

RIGHT MEDIAL, LEFT LATERAL

Figure 3.76 Mild anterior impingement of the right ankle demonstrating focal uptake on both the tibial and talar sides of the joint margin. There is also evidence of right Achilles tendon enthesopathy.

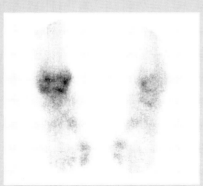

ANTERIOR

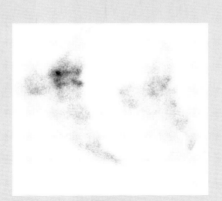

RIGHT LATERAL, LEFT MEDIAL

Figure 3.77 Severe right ankle anterior impingement with more extensive joint margin involvement.

Posterior impingement syndrome (Fig. 3.78)

The posterior impingement syndrome is clinically manifested by pain behind the ankle joint occurring with plantar flexion of the ankle. Hyperextension of the ankle occurs with kicking and can be very important in classic dance, where discomfort will occur with the *en pointe* position. Predisposing factors include a prominent posterior process of the talus and the presence of an os trigonum. Soft tissue causes include synovitis and a ganglion.

Other ankle impingements

Following trauma, bony spurs commonly develop at the medial and lateral malleoli and these may impinge on the adjacent talus. These conditions can also be identified by focal increased uptake occurring at the site of bony abutment.

Figure 3.78 Posterior impingement with focal uptake in the posterior process of the left talus. Note also the left first tarsometatarsal arthritis.

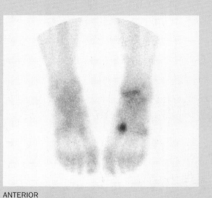

ANTERIOR

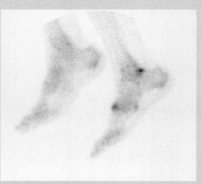

RIGHT MEDIAL, LEFT LATERAL

Tarsal coalition (Figs 3.79–3.81)

This condition is present when there is a developmental osseous, cartilaginous, or fibrous union between tarsal bones. The commonest coalitions are talocalcaneal and calcaneonavicular with calcaneocuboid coalition rarely seen. They may be bilateral. This condition causes stiffness and foot pain in the tarsal region and usually presents in the second and third decades.

The diagnosis is initially established with plain films and CT scanning. A bone scan will show increased uptake corresponding with the fibrous or cartilaginous site of coalition. This condition must always be kept in mind when increase in uptake is demonstrated in the subtalar region in an adolescent.

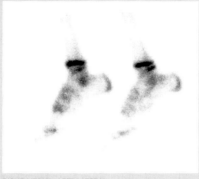

RIGHT MEDIAL, LEFT LATERAL

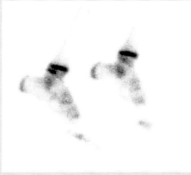

RIGHT LATERAL, LEFT MEDIAL

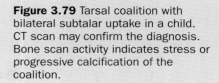

Figure 3.79 Tarsal coalition with bilateral subtalar uptake in a child. CT scan may confirm the diagnosis. Bone scan activity indicates stress or progressive calcification of the coalition.

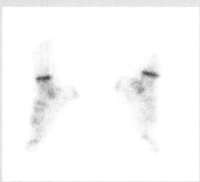

BLOOD POOL FROGLEG

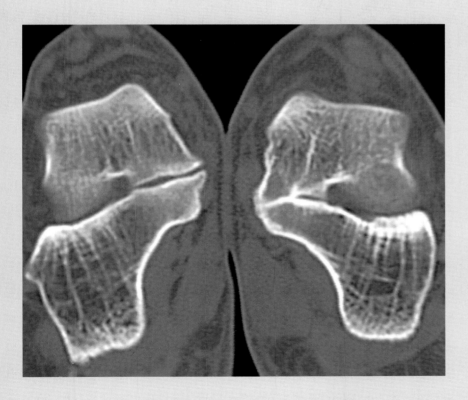

Figure 3.80 CT scan shows fibrous or cartilagenous coalition on the right side and partial osseous coalition across the left middle subtalar joint.

Figure 3.81 Tarsal coalition with bilateral uptake in the talonavicular and calcaneocuboid joints.

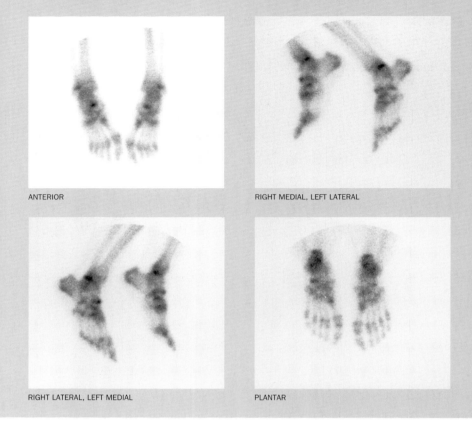

ANTERIOR

RIGHT MEDIAL, LEFT LATERAL

RIGHT LATERAL, LEFT MEDIAL

PLANTAR

Arthritis and synovitis (Figs 3.82–3.84)

The diagnosis of arthritis or synovitis in the ankle or foot depends on localising the uptake to the articular surfaces, usually involving both sides of a joint. If only one side of the joint is involved, then osteochondral fracture needs to be considered. The blood pool images may aid in differentiation. In arthritis the blood pool changes are usually more diffuse. The diagnosis is relatively easy in large joints such as the knee, but in small joints in the tarsal region, the distinction may not be possible, as individual bones cannot be clearly resolved. For this reason, midtarsal arthritis, whether traumatic synovitis or frank osteoarthritis, may be difficult to distinguish from changes in bone, such as a fracture.

Subtalar joint arthritis can be difficult to differentiate from ankle joint problems clinically but has a characteristic appearance on bone scan, allowing this differentiation to be made. A bone scan shows a linear band of increased uptake of isotope running obliquely along the line of the subtalar joint and is best seen in the lateral or medial views.

Traumatic synovitis is usually the result of joint sprain. This condition manifests as a diffuse increase in uptake throughout the joint and these changes may make identification of an osteochondral fracture difficult, particularly if imaged very early in the course of the injury. This differentiation may need to be made by CT scanning or, ideally, by MRI.

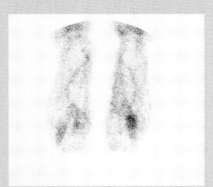

BLOOD POOL PLANTAR

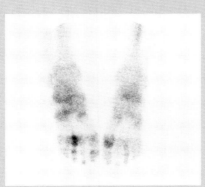

ANTERIOR

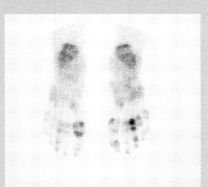

PLANTAR

Figure 3.82 Inflammatory arthropathy due to psoriasis. The early view demonstrates a marked increase in blood flow throughout the third toes bilaterally. Delayed images show periarticular increase in uptake in these toes, most marked in the right third MTP joint. Low-grade arthritis is also seen in the first toes and in the tarsal joints.

Figure 3.83 Inflammatory arthropathy due to gout. There is increased uptake in multiple joints including the ankles, tarsal joints and in both first metatarsophalangeal joints. Note the uptake in the tophi in the Achilles tendons and at the right Achilles insertion.

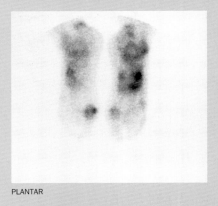

PLANTAR

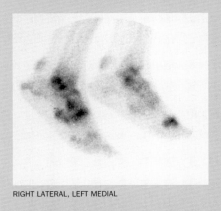

RIGHT LATERAL, LEFT MEDIAL

Figure 3.84 Right subtalar joint arthritis following trauma. Uptake is seen in the line of the subtalar joint.

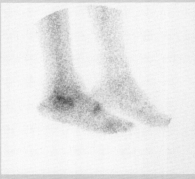

BLOOD POOL RIGHT LATERAL, LEFT MEDIAL

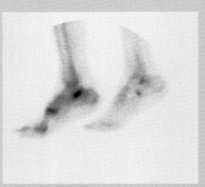

RIGHT MEDIAL, LEFT LATERAL

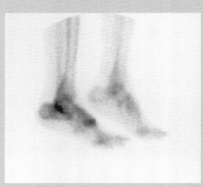

RIGHT LATERAL, LEFT MEDIAL

Lisfranc fracture dislocation and sagittal diastasis (Figs 3.85–3.91)

The diagnosis of this injury is important to establish as considerable discomfort and disability occur when only minor bony change may be present. This injury is often difficult to diagnose using plain films due to superimposition of bones at the tarsometatarsal joints. A plantodorsal plain film view can be used to help display the bony surfaces at the tarsometatarsal joints. Subtle injury can be impossible to detect and other imaging methods are usually employed.

The key structure involved in this injury is the Lisfranc ligament running from the medial aspect of the base of the second metatarsal to the adjacent lateral aspect of the medial cuneiform. This is a potential site of weakness as there is no ligamentous stabilisation between the first and second metatarsal bases. Following midfoot plantarflexion, the Lisfranc ligament may be ruptured. This ligament is the key to stability of the tarsometatarsal joints, and injury to this ligament allows disruption extending transversely across the tarsometatarsal joints, with either a divergent or homolateral deformity resulting.

Landing on the ball of the foot with a twisting movement may also injure the Lisfranc ligament, but the shearing force extends in the sagittal plane, rather than across the foot, disrupting the articulation between the medial and middle cuneiforms. This is a sagittal diastasis.

Consequently, there are two patterns of injury seen on bone scan following disruption of the Lisfranc ligament. The flow study, early and delayed views show increased blood flow and uptake of isotope in a line across the tarsometatarsal junction with a Lisfranc fracture dislocation and along the sagittal plane with a sagittal diastasis. Some injuries are confined only to the area of the Lisfranc ligament.

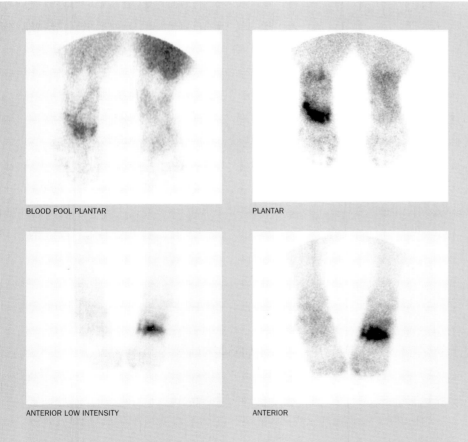

BLOOD POOL PLANTAR

PLANTAR

ANTERIOR LOW INTENSITY

ANTERIOR

Figure 3.85 Lisfranc injury. Fracture/dislocation showing intense uptake on both the early and delayed views in all the left tarsometatarsal joints.

Figure 3.86 Tarsometatarsal fracture/dislocations. A plantodorsal X-ray view of the tarsometatarsal region will show the joint spaces and help define the resultant deformity. This is an example of a homolateral deformity where all metatarsal heads are subluxed laterally. In a divergent deformity, the first metatarsal will be displaced medially and the other metatarsals laterally. Note the fragments avulsed by the Lisfranc ligament.

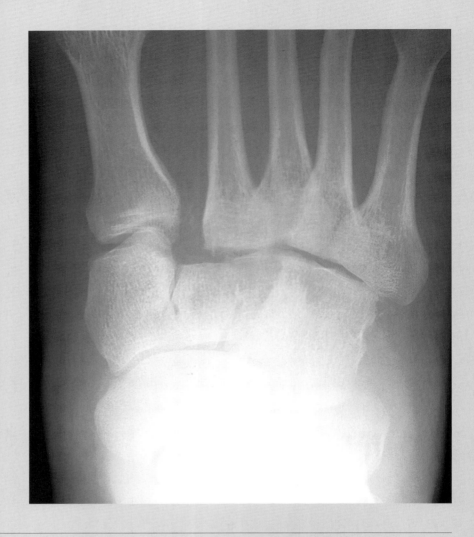

Figure 3.87 CT of a Lisfranc fracture/dislocation. This is a classic example showing fractures of the bases of the second, third and fourth metatarsals and the distal articular surface of the cuboid. In practice, plain film changes of a Lisfranc fracture/dislocation are difficult to detect and a bone scan is usually required to establish the diagnosis. Having established the diagnosis with a bone scan, a CT scan will demonstrate the extent of the bone injury, which is invariably more extensive than expected.

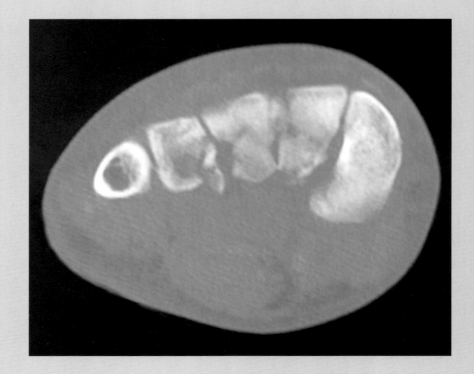

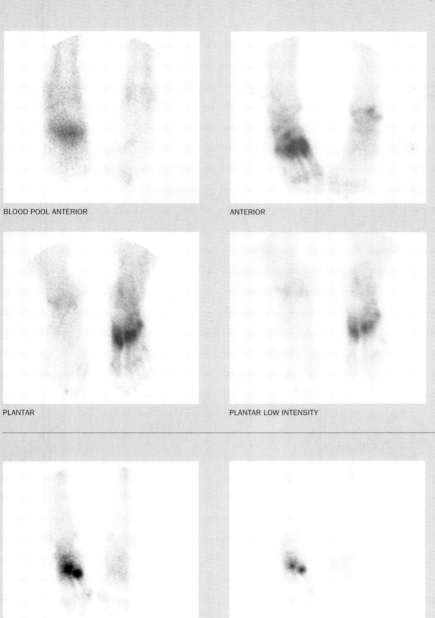

Figure 3.88 Lisfranc injury with involvement more on the medial side of the right tarsometatarsal joint line.

BLOOD POOL ANTERIOR

ANTERIOR

PLANTAR

PLANTAR LOW INTENSITY

Figure 3.89 Lisfranc injury confined to the first and second tarsometatarsal joints, sparing the lateral joints. There is focal uptake in the metatarsal heads, indicating fracture.

ANTERIOR

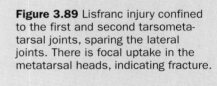

ANTERIOR LOW INTENSITY

PLANTAR

PLANTAR LOW INTENSITY

Figure 3.90 (right, below and top of opposite page) Rupture of the Lisfranc ligament may also result in a sagittal diastasis. A small avulsion is shown on plain films between the medial cuneiform and the base of the second metatarsal. A CT scan shows separation of the first and second rays on the left side. MRI shows the extensive associated oedema.

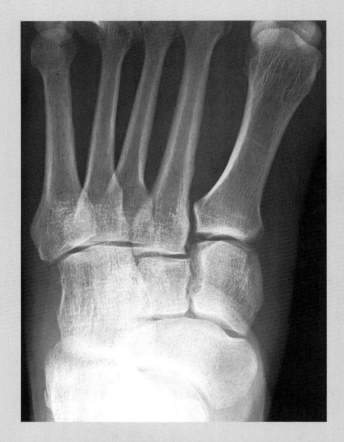

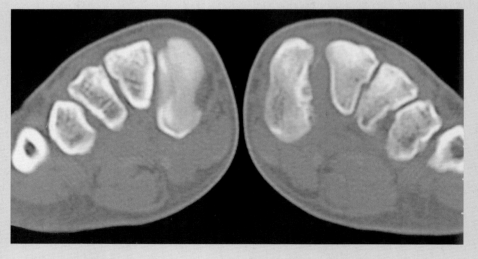

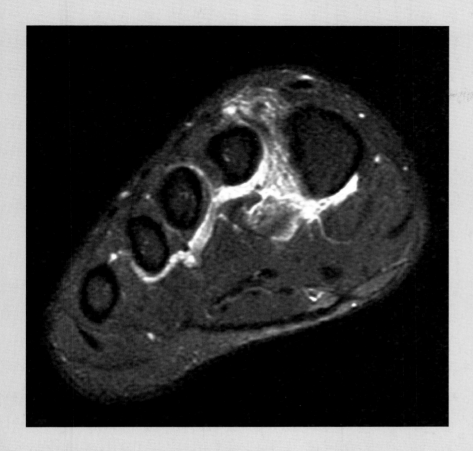

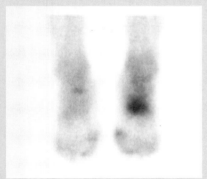

ANTERIOR

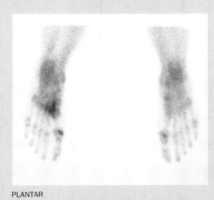

PLANTAR

Figure 3.91 Sagittal diastasis with uptake in the line of the left medial intercuneiform joint.

The sesamoids (Figs 3.92–3.96)

Sesamoiditis is a condition characterised by pain beneath the head of the first metatarsal and is seen commonly in ballet and gymnastics. Sesamoiditis is an overuse injury caused by repetitive stress producing ischaemic changes. Injury to the sesamoids can also be due to direct trauma causing a fracture or a stress fracture without ischaemic change.

A bipartite sesamoid may be confused with a fracture, when looking at sesamoids on plain films. This is a common dilemma. An uncomplicated bipartite deformity will not show an increased uptake of isotope. Occasionally, disruption of the bipartite configuration can occur as a result of trauma.

Bone scans are useful in establishing a diagnosis, particularly when the plain film changes are equivocal. The plantar and true medial views demonstrate a focus of uptake coinciding with either the medial or lateral sesamoid.

Frank fracture of a sesamoid shows an increase in both blood flow and uptake. Sesamoiditis, being ischaemic, is less likely to show an increase in blood flow and will show low-grade increase in uptake.

Figure 3.92 Right medial sesamoiditis in a child. Note that the true medial view demonstrates more clearly that the uptake is in the sesamoid bone beneath the first MTP joint and not in the joint. As is often the case, the anterior view is normal. Note also the physeal activity in multiple bones.

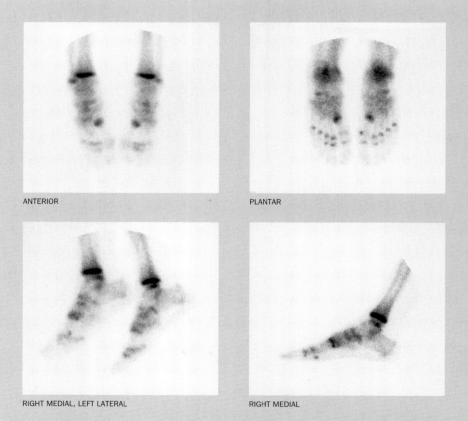

ANTERIOR

PLANTAR

RIGHT MEDIAL, LEFT LATERAL

RIGHT MEDIAL

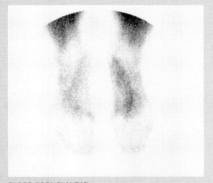

BLOOD POOL PLANTAR

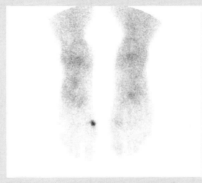

PLANTAR

Figure 3.93 Left medial sesamoiditis.

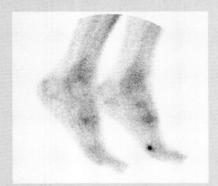

RIGHT LATERAL, LEFT MEDIAL

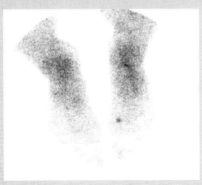

PLANTAR

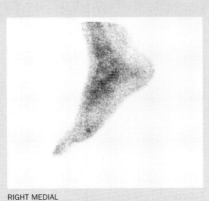

RIGHT MEDIAL

Figure 3.94 Right lateral sesamoiditis.

Figure 3.95 A tangential view of the sesamoids demonstrates changes of sesamoiditis in the medial sesamoid. These changes are typical of an avascular process, with sclerosis, fragmentation and compression.

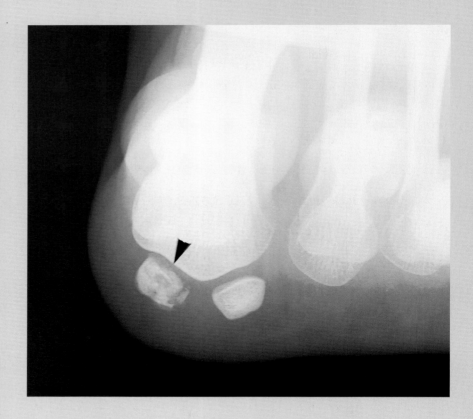

Figure 3.96 Bone spur imitating sesamoiditis. The plantar view shows focal uptake at the right first MTP joint; however, the right medial view shows the activity to be dorsal rather than plantar. X-ray confirmed a prominent dorsal osteophyte.

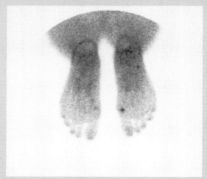

PLANTAR

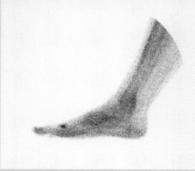

RIGHT MEDIAL

Morton's neuroma

The bone scan is normal in this condition.

Painful os peroneum syndrome (POP)

An os peroneum is a sesamoid bone in the peroneus longus tendon, protecting the tendon as it curves around the lateral border of the cuboid. This accessory ossicle may become traumatised and can cause lateral foot pain. It is frequently associated with peroneus longus tendinosis. The bone scan characteristically shows a localised increase in uptake.

Reflex sympathetic dystrophy (Figs 3.97–3.99)

This interesting condition often involves the foot and ankle following seemingly trivial trauma. The ankle and foot become painful and swollen with tenderness, vasomotor changes, hyperaesthesia and considerable disability.

As in this condition elsewhere, the bone-scan changes are seen before the radiological changes appear. The changes are also seen to persist for a period after clinical recovery. Characteristically, the blood pool phase shows a diffuse increase in blood flow with an increase in uptake seen in the delayed images in a periarticular distribution. Other patterns of decreased flow and uptake have been described.

In the authors' experience, regional involvement is commonly seen as a post-traumatic event, with regional increase in uptake on both the blood pool and delayed images.

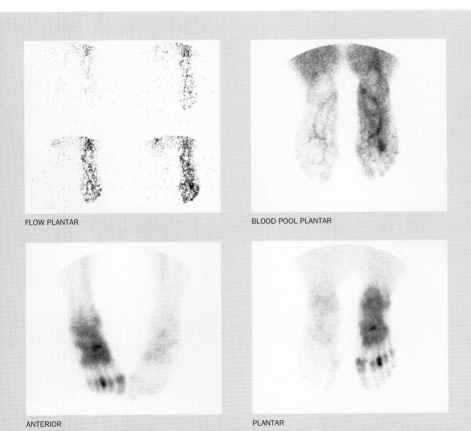

FLOW PLANTAR

BLOOD POOL PLANTAR

ANTERIOR

PLANTAR

Figure 3.97 Reflex sympathetic dystrophy showing a diffuse increase in tracer activity throughout the right foot on the flow, blood pool and delayed images, especially in a periarticular distribution. This is superimposed on focal inflammation in the right third MTP joint.

Figure 3.98 Regional osteoporosis. There is regional hypervascularity and increased uptake diffusely throughout the left mid and hind foot, but sparing the forefoot. This occurred 3 months after the left fibular fracture and ankle trauma.

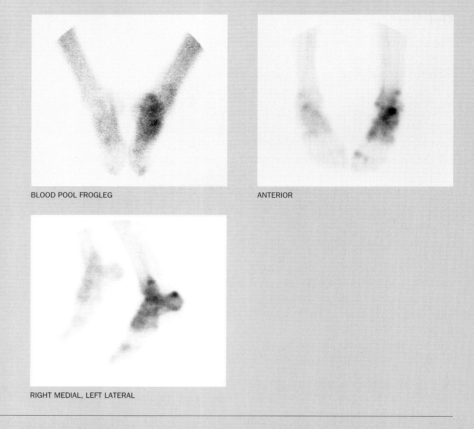

BLOOD POOL FROGLEG   ANTERIOR

RIGHT MEDIAL, LEFT LATERAL

Figure 3.99 Regional osteoporosis involving the tarsal bones, sparing the calcaneum and forefoot. Both early and delayed uptake are increased.

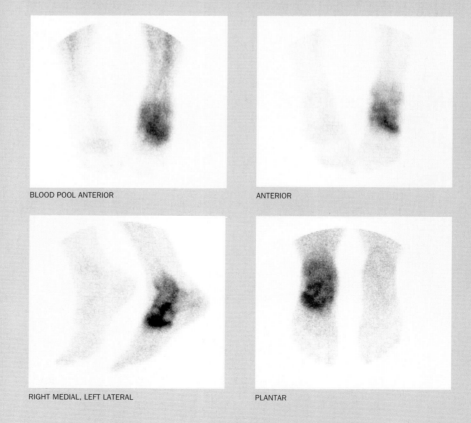

BLOOD POOL ANTERIOR   ANTERIOR

RIGHT MEDIAL, LEFT LATERAL   PLANTAR

The heel

Bone scanning contributes to the diagnosis of both bony and soft tissue processes occurring at the heel. In the elite athlete, Achilles tendinitis and plantar fasciitis are extremely common causes of heel pain. Bone scans can be helpful in the diagnosis of both acute and chronic calcaneal fractures.

Calcaneal fractures (Figs 3.100–3.103)

Calcaneal fractures may result from acute trauma and a bone scan can be helpful if plain films are equivocal. Some fractures, such as a fracture of the sustentaculum tali, may be difficult to demonstrate on plain films. Stress fractures of the calcaneum are not commonly seen in athletes and are usually seen as insufficiency fractures in the older age group. Calcaneal stress fractures from overuse are traditionally seen in military recruits. The bone scan typically shows a diffuse increase in uptake throughout the calcaneum. It is often necessary to reduce the intensity of the image markedly and then a linear area of greater activity can be demonstrated.

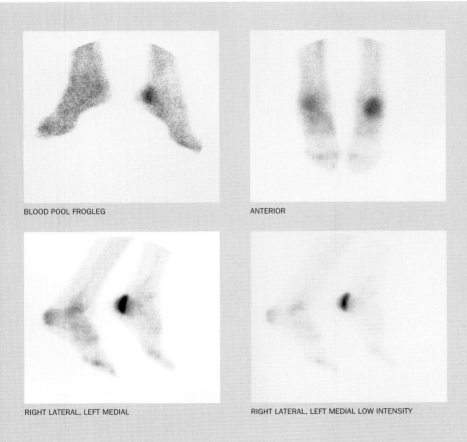

BLOOD POOL FROGLEG

ANTERIOR

RIGHT LATERAL, LEFT MEDIAL

RIGHT LATERAL, LEFT MEDIAL LOW INTENSITY

Figure 3.100 Vertical fracture of the calcaneum. Increased blood flow and linear increase in uptake vertically in the left calcaneum.
Note: (1) Reducing the intensity of the image highlights the linear nature of the uptake. (2) The normal bone posterior to the fracture line indicates that the uptake is not due to Achilles avulsion fracture. (3) The medial views are essential to exclude the uptake being in the talus.

Figure 3.101 An insufficiency
fracture. The calcaneum is
demineralised and a stress fracture
has been caused by normal stress
on abnormal bone.

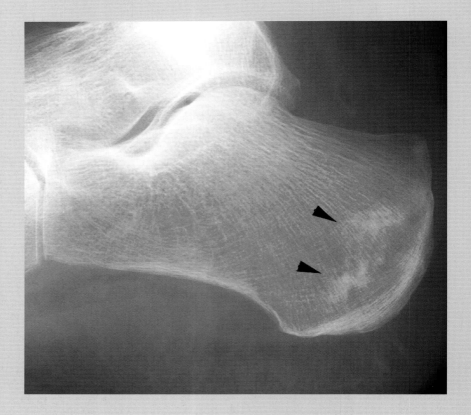

Figure 3.102 Fracture in the
calcaneum close to the subtalar
joint. Note that the increase in
uptake stops at the subtalar joint but
flares into the right calcaneum.
Because of the intensity of uptake, it
is difficult to obtain one image
showing all of the detail. Images at
different intensities help to alleviate
this problem. Note also the fractures
in the base of the left first
metatarsal and shaft of the left
second metatarsal.

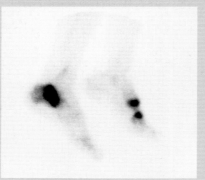

RIGHT LATERAL, LEFT MEDIAL

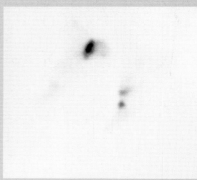

RIGHT MEDIAL, LEFT LATERAL

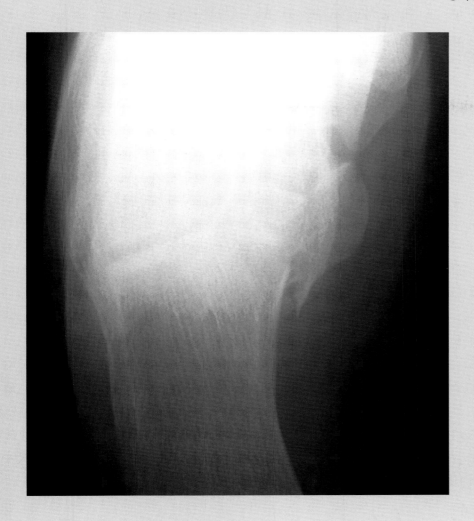

Figure 3.103 A fracture of the sustentaculum tali is demonstrated by a Harris-Beath view.

Achilles tendinosis and associated conditions (Figs 3.104–3.111)

These conditions are some of the commonest problems encountered in the elite track-and-field athlete. The diagnosis is established clinically, but further investigations are required to ascertain whether Achilles tendinosis is focal or diffuse, whether there is a tear in the tendon, whether there are changes in the paratenon and to help assess whether these changes contribute significantly to the symptoms. Associated conditions, such as insertional enthesopathy, retrocalcaneal bursitis, tendoAchilles bursitis and pre-Achilles fat pad changes may also be present. Imaging is initially by plain films and other methods are then used, depending on the clinical suspicions.

Insertional enthesopathy can be seen on bone scan or MRI. The extent of the tendinosis, changes in the fat pad, tendon tears, paratenon thickening and bursitis can be imaged by MRI or by ultrasound. The accuracy of ultrasound is dependent on a competent musculoskeletal operator.

Enthesopathy at the insertion of the Achilles tendon

The flow study may show an increase in blood flow if the process is advanced, or it may be normal. In the delayed films, a focus of increased uptake of isotope in the calcaneum adjacent to the Achilles insertion is indicative of enthesopathy.

Retrocalcaneal bursitis

Retrocalcaneal bursitis may develop independently of a full-blown Haglund's syndrome and the bone scan shows a focus of uptake on early and delayed views in the calcaneum adjacent to the retrocalcaneal sulcus.

Haglund's syndrome

When the bursal protuberance of the calcaneum is prominent, friction may occur between the protuberance and the adjacent Achilles tendon, producing tendinosis and retrocalcaneal bursitis. A bursa superficial to the lower end of the Achilles tendon, the tendoAchilles bursa, is usually also involved. These changes make up Haglund's syndrome. The diagnosis may be established on plain films, but can be suspected on scans performed for other reasons, if there is increased uptake on the posterosuperior aspect of the calcaneal tuberosity.

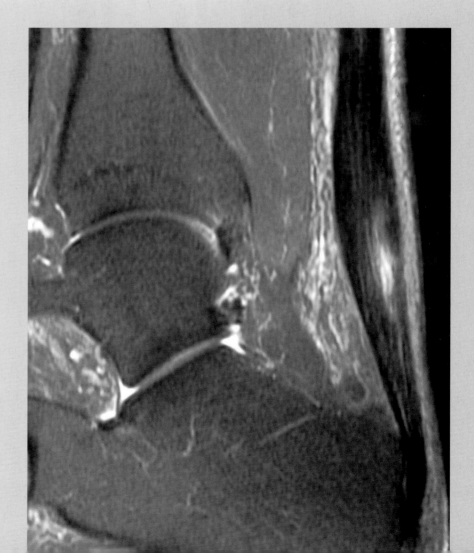

Figure 3.104 (right and opposite page) Achilles tendinopathy. The sagittal MRI image shows extensive high signal in a swollen Achilles tendon. The axial image demonstrates a tear (arrow) complicating extensive tendinosis.

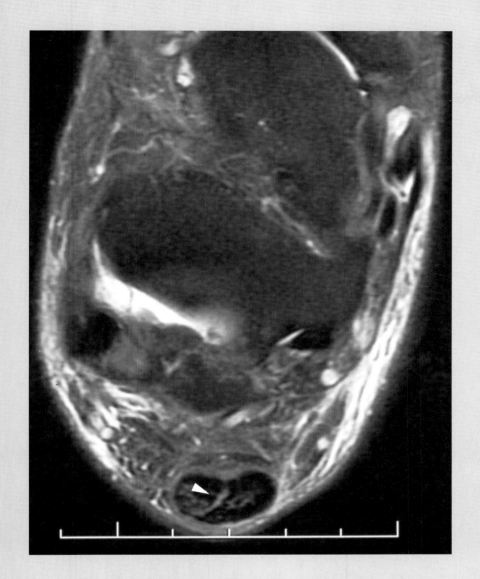

Figure 3.105 Bilateral Achilles enthesopathy. Increased blood flow, blood pool and delayed uptake at the site of left Achilles tendon insertion into the middle third of the posterior aspect of the left calcaneum. Low-grade similar injury is evident in the right calcaneum.

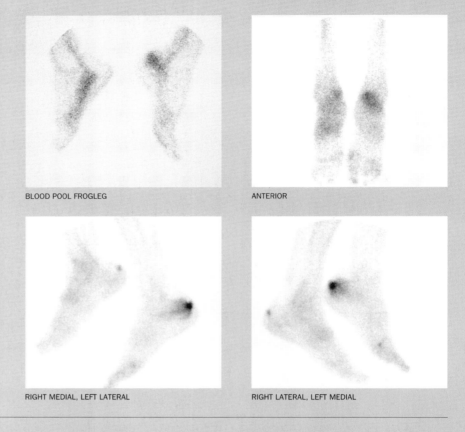

BLOOD POOL FROGLEG

ANTERIOR

RIGHT MEDIAL, LEFT LATERAL

RIGHT LATERAL, LEFT MEDIAL

Figure 3.106 Right Achilles enthesopathy. The inflammation is more widespread than the previous case.

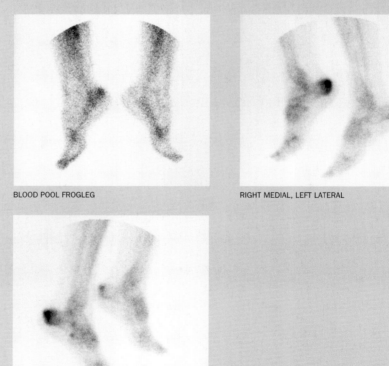

BLOOD POOL FROGLEG

RIGHT MEDIAL, LEFT LATERAL

RIGHT LATERAL, LEFT MEDIAL

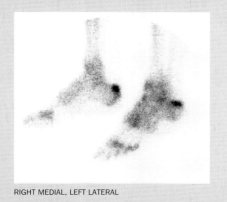
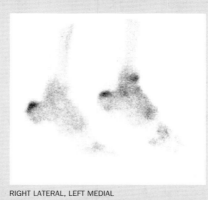

RIGHT MEDIAL, LEFT LATERAL

RIGHT LATERAL, LEFT MEDIAL

Figure 3.107 Achilles enthesopathy and retrocalcaneal bursitis. The increase in uptake extends to the superior surface of the calcaneum due to a combination of Achilles insertion enthesopathy and retrocalcaneal bursitis.

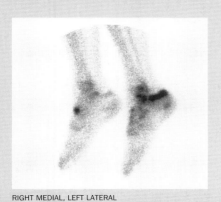
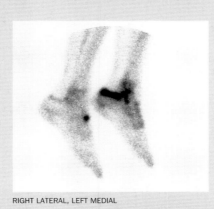

RIGHT MEDIAL, LEFT LATERAL

RIGHT LATERAL, LEFT MEDIAL

Figure 3.108 Retrocalcaneal bursitis. There is intense uptake along the superior surface of the left calcaneum with minimal increase in uptake at the same site on the right.

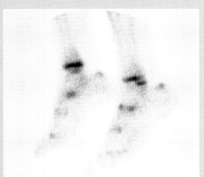

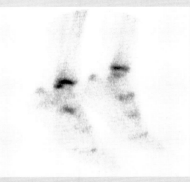

RIGHT MEDIAL, LEFT LATERAL

RIGHT LATERAL, LEFT MEDIAL

Figure 3.109 Haglund's syndrome. Mildly increased uptake can be demonstrated in the prominent superior surface of the calcaneum (Haglund's lump) where the Achilles tendon impinges.

Figure 3.110 Haglund's syndrome has four components: Achilles tendinopathy, retrocalcaneal bursitis, tendoAchilles bursitis and (usually) a prominent bursal protrusion. In this X-ray, the protrusion shows irregularity and possible erosion.

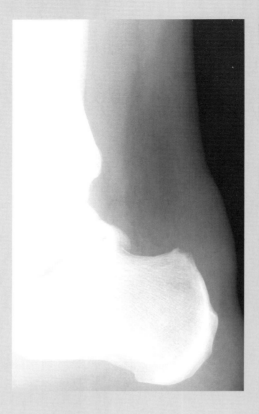

Figure 3.111 Longstanding Achilles enthesopathies and Achilles tendinitis with calcification in the left Achilles tendon, intense uptake throughout the insertion sites and arthritis in the left midfoot.

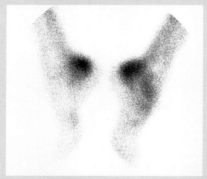

BLOOD POOL FROGLEG

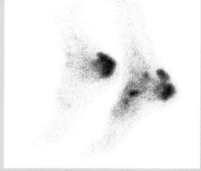

RIGHT MEDIAL, LEFT LATERAL

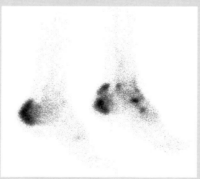

RIGHT LATERAL, LEFT MEDIAL

Plantar fasciitis (Figs 3.112–3.117)

Frogleg early views may be normal, may show a diffuse increase in vascularity along the sole, or show a focus of hyperaemia at the insertion. The delayed images usually show the enthesopathy with a focus of increased uptake of isotope at the calcaneal attachment of the plantar fascia. If the pathology is confined to soft tissue, the delayed image may be normal.

There may be continuous enthesopathy involving the insertion of the plantar fascia and the Achilles tendon. A plantar spur may develop from repetitive traction at the calcaneal insertion. Fracture of a spur does not cause increased uptake in the body of the calcaneum.

Enthesopathies may also occur at the insertion of the short plantar ligament and at the distal plantar fascia insertions.

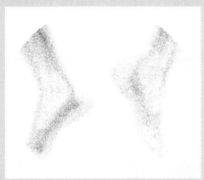

BLOOD POOL FROGLEG

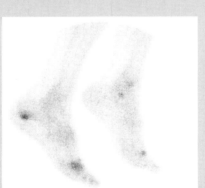

RIGHT LATERAL, LEFT MEDIAL

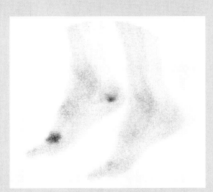

RIGHT MEDIAL, LEFT LATERAL

Figure 3.112 Plantar fasciitis and enthesopathy. Increased blood pool activity along the sole of the right foot. The delayed images show only a small focus of uptake in the inferior surface of the right calcaneum. This case shows inflammation both in the soft tissue of the plantar fascia and at the insertion into the calcaneum. Note also the arthritis in both first MTP joints.

Figure 3.113 Plantar fasciitis. There is increased blood pool activity along the right plantar fascia but no significant increase in activity at the calcaneal insertion, demonstrating plantar fasciitis without enthesopathy.

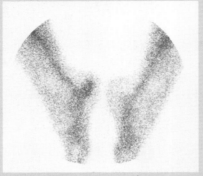

BLOOD POOL FROGLEG

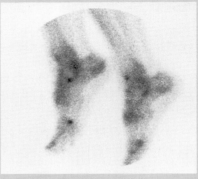

RIGHT MEDIAL, LEFT LATERAL

Figure 3.114 Ultrasound demonstrates swelling of the plantar fascia and disruption of fibrils indicates a partial tear (arrow).

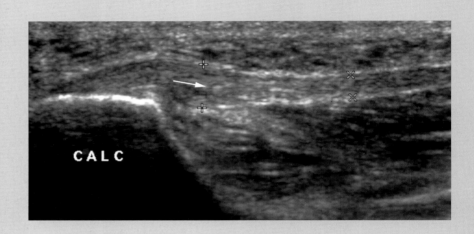

Figure 3.115 Plantar fascia enthesopathy with increased blood pool activity and delayed uptake only at the insertion site in the right calcaneum inferiorly. No soft tissue inflammation is seen along the sole.

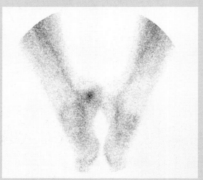

BLOOD POOL FROGLEG

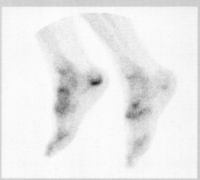

RIGHT MEDIAL, LEFT LATERAL

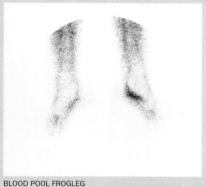

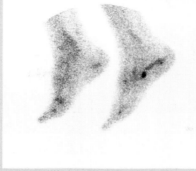

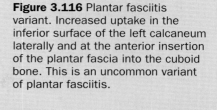

Figure 3.116 Plantar fasciitis variant. Increased uptake in the inferior surface of the left calcaneum laterally and at the anterior insertion of the plantar fascia into the cuboid bone. This is an uncommon variant of plantar fasciitis.

BLOOD POOL FROGLEG

RIGHT MEDIAL, LEFT LATERAL

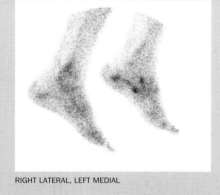

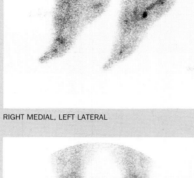

RIGHT LATERAL, LEFT MEDIAL

PLANTAR

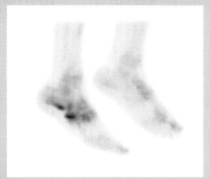

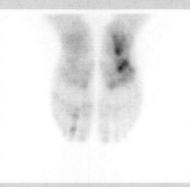

Figure 3.117 Short plantar ligament enthesopathy. The focal increase in uptake of isotope in the plantar surface of the right calcaneum is at the origin of the short plantar ligament. There is also uptake at its cuboid insertion. This unusual case shows evidence of disruption of the short plantar ligament with tear at its insertions at each end.

RIGHT LATERAL, LEFT MEDIAL

PLANTAR

Trauma to the calcaneal apophysis (Fig 3.118)

Prior to fusion of the calcaneal apophysis, trauma to the apophysis may result in injury to the growth plate. There is increased blood pool activity and delayed uptake in the unfused apophysis, resulting in asymmetry. This bone scan appearance is consistent with a fracture through the growth plate. It is best demonstrated in the frogleg position.

Figure 3.118 Trauma to the calcaneal physis. There is a focal increase in blood flow and bony uptake in the left posterior calcaneal physis. The blood pool image is often the most helpful in making this diagnosis. Simultaneous imaging of the physes in the same anatomical position can best be obtained in the medials/frogleg position. We believe this is a fracture through the growth plate and is the condition frequently termed Sever's disease.

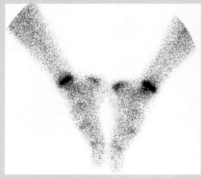
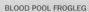

BLOOD POOL FROGLEG

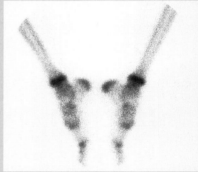

FROGLEG

There are many causes of exercise-induced pain in the lower leg. These include bone stress and stress fractures, periosteal reaction, compartment syndromes, tendinitis, muscle tears and rarer causes such as muscle hernias, nerve entrapment, vascular insufficiency (which may be due to arterial disease or vessel entrapment), deep venous thrombosis (which may be effort-induced), ruptured popliteal cyst, sciatica and spinal stenosis.

The confusion of terminologies

Exercise-induced leg pain is a common complaint amongst athletes. The subject is complex and confused due to the large number of causes, the occurrence of more than one cause at the one time and the use of the term 'shin splints'.

To some people, the term 'shin splints' refers to all exercise-induced pain in the leg and to others it is confined to pain occurring anteriorly, while still others use the term to infer 'medial tibial stress syndrome'. 'Shin splints' was first coined by Mubarak et al. in 1982 to describe exercise-induced pain on the posteromedial aspect of the tibia. Still further confusion then arose due to attempts to associate the term 'shin splints' with a particular pathological process. Holder and Michael in 1984 proposed that shin splints produced a specific appearance on bone scan, with linear uptake demonstrated along the tibial shaft only on delayed bone scan images. Subsequent biopsy studies by Detmer have shown this to be an oversimplification.

Detmer's paper, 'Chronic shin splints', in 1986 classified 'medial tibial stress syndrome' into three types, that are differentiated by which anatomical structure is involved.

Detmer's three entities are:

- type I, where the primary problem is the bone itself, including stress fractures and bone stress reaction or tibial microfracture. Within this category are type I-A (focal lesion) and type I-B (more diffuse and often vertical linear);
- type II, where the symptoms are at the periosteal/fascial junction just adjacent to the bone;
- type III, where the symptoms are even more posterior, localising to the soft muscular tissues behind the tibia.

In our experience this classification corresponds with the three bone-scan appearances commonly seen in the investigation of tibial shaft pain:

1. stress fracture (focal or linear)—Detmer type I;
2. periosteal reaction—Detmer type II;
3. normal scan—Detmer type III.

Type I is injury at the cortical level, due to bone stress. The athlete will have tenderness on palpation over the tibial margin and this may be localised (type I-A) or extend for a varying length along the shaft for distances of up to 6 to 10 cm (type I-B). As with bone stress and stress fractures elsewhere, plain films are characteristically normal in the acute case, but may show thickening of the cortex and periosteal new bone, or occasionally a fracture line in the more chronic injury. The bone scan shows the typical appearance of bone stress or stress fracture.

Type II is an injury at the interface between periosteum and fascia. Detmer found an increased incidence in runners (especially sprinters and hurdlers) and in jumping sports (gymnasts, dancers, and basketball). On palpation, tenderness is maximal at the junction of the periosteum and the fascia. The site of involvement is most commonly seen in the middle and distal thirds of the tibia, usually beginning about 5 to 7 cm above the medial malleolus and extending 6 to 8 cm or occasionally much higher. Imaging of this condition requires an understanding of the process.

In the acute stages, the posteromedial angle of the tibial shaft is stressed by traction of the fascia that attaches at the angle. Traction is produced by the action of the soleus and/or the flexor digitorum longus. Changes of stress occur in the periosteum and changes of periosteal reaction are found on biopsy. At this stage the bone scan shows evidence of the periosteal reaction. Holder's description appeared to hold true and is in agreement with our experience. Some authors suggest there is a continuum from periosteal reaction to subperiosteal bone stress and stress fracture. This remains controversial.

If the periosteum becomes detached and reattachment does not occur, the condition becomes intractable. Symptoms will recur promptly after periods of rest. In Detmer's operative series, fat was consistently found between the periosteum and the underlying bone, without evidence of periosteal reaction. Although the periosteum is disengaged, it remains innervated and it is suggested that the condition remains painful due to continued fascial traction on the elevated periosteum. There are no good data as to how often this occurs. In these chronic cases the bone scan may fail to demonstrate any changes. Consequently, in spite of severe symptoms in chronic Detmer type II cases, imaging may be normal. It is therefore possible that typical chronic symptoms and a normal scan may indicate an adverse prognosis. Plain films should still be obtained to ensure that there are no unexpected pathological changes present.

To further complicate the concept of 'shin splints', Zwas in 1987 described anterolateral diffuse periosteal uptake as shin splints. Because of the confusion associated with the term, it is probably best avoided. The descriptive term of 'periosteal reaction' may be preferable.

Type III refers to a process involving muscle in its fascial compartment, a so-called compartment syndrome. The deep posterior compartment syndrome can present with posteromedial exercise-induced pain. Tenderness is elicited in the muscular soft tissues posterior to the periosteal/fascial junction and deep within the leg. Plain films and bone scans are normal.

In summary, Detmer demonstrated that bone scans are reliable in the diagnosis of bone stress fractures and acute periosteal reaction, but are often normal in compartment syndromes and chronic periosteal traction.

Tips on technique

A three-phase study should be performed with the early views obtained over the region of maximal pain and tenderness. Extra blood pool images of adjacent areas and orthogonal views may be necessary.

Delayed images of the lower legs should be obtained in the anterior, lateral, medial and posterior projections. As with all imaging in sports medicine, joints above and below the site of pain must be included, with anterior views of the knees, ankles and feet being obtained. Extra lateral or medial views of the knees and ankles are sometimes required. The study must be tailored to the clinical picture and modified as required, depending on the results of the initial standard images (Fig. 4.1).

Figure 4.1 Standard views.

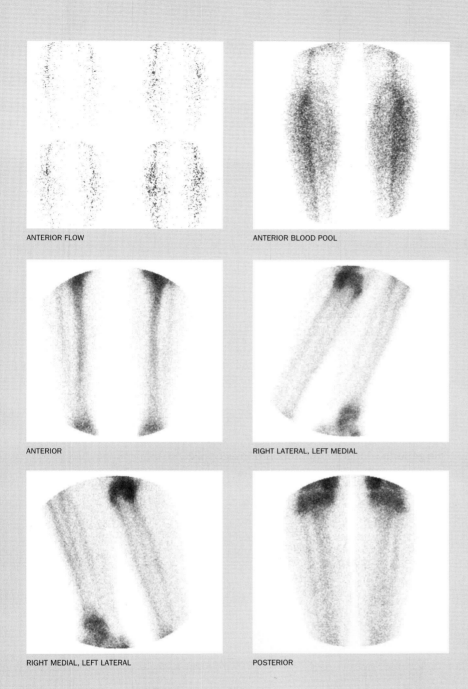

ANTERIOR FLOW

ANTERIOR BLOOD POOL

ANTERIOR

RIGHT LATERAL, LEFT MEDIAL

RIGHT MEDIAL, LEFT LATERAL

POSTERIOR

Bone stress and fractures of the tibia and fibula

Bone scan appearance

In the acute phase, the flow and blood pool images typically show increased vascularity, the intensity of which is often related to the severity of the fracture. The delayed images show focal increase in uptake at the site of the fracture.

As healing progresses, the flow phase is the first to return to normal, followed by the blood pool images. The delayed focal uptake resolves slowly over weeks to months, the duration being at least partially related to the initial severity of the fracture and the degree of callus formation.

There is little role for repeat imaging of the stress fracture, unless symptoms persist or recur.

As with many other processes, authors have staged stress fractures with two frequently quoted classifications being those of Matin (I–V), and Zwas (I–IV). It is not our practice to report a numerical stage of the fracture because of confusion arising from the variation between classifications. The authors prefer to classify them as low-, medium- or high-grade fractures.

Fractures (Figs 4.2–4.29)

Fractures can be due to acute trauma or the progression of bone stress to tissue failure. Acute fractures of the tibia and fibula occur occasionally in sport, but are rarely subtle and do not usually require a bone scan. If the X-ray is normal and symptoms and signs are suggestive of a fracture, then a bone scan should be performed to confirm or exclude an occult fracture.

Stress fractures occur commonly in the tibia and fibula, particularly in runners. Bone stress occurs in many sites and the sites described by various authors reflect their referral patterns. Common sites include:

*   the medial tibial condyle parallel to the articular surface of the plateau. This was said to be the commonest site of tibial stress fracture;
*   the proximal tibia posteriorly, just below the level of the tibial tuberosity. This is seen in young runners;
*   the anterior tibial cortex in jumping sports and in ballet;
*   the posteromedial aspect of the middle third of the distal tibia;
*   the distal tibial metaphysis;
*   the distal tibial shaft in a spiral or linear pattern;
*   the shaft of the fibula at muscle attachments;
*   the distal fibula just above the level of the distal tibiofibular joint. This is commonly seen in recreational long-distance runners;
*   the neck of the fibula.

Stress fractures in the proximal shaft and anterior cortex are often slow to recover, with a greater risk of progression to a complete fracture. Consequently, early diagnosis is important, and a bone scan should be obtained early in the patient's management.

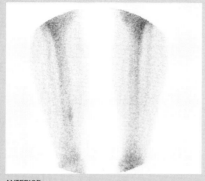
ANTERIOR

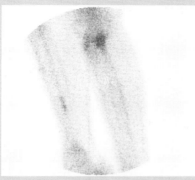
RIGHT MEDIAL, LEFT LATERAL

Figure 4.2 Minimal focal increase in uptake in the posteromedial border of the right tibia due to stress reaction or low-grade stress fracture.

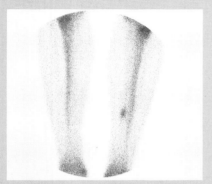
ANTERIOR

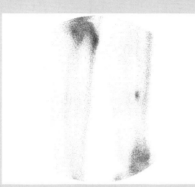
RIGHT LATERAL, LEFT MEDIAL

Figure 4.3 Low-grade stress fracture of the left tibia.

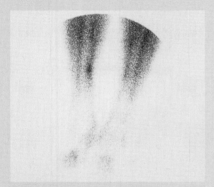
ANTERIOR BLOOD POOL

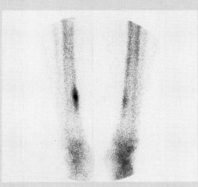
ANTERIOR

Figure 4.4 Medium grade right tibial stress fracture and mild left tibial stress reaction—the left was asymptomatic. Note the focal vascularity on the blood pool image.

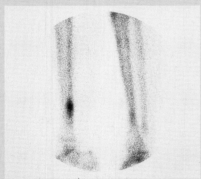
RIGHT MEDIAL, LEFT LATERAL

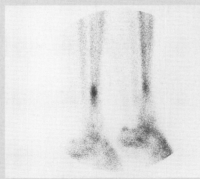
RIGHT LATERAL, LEFT MEDIAL

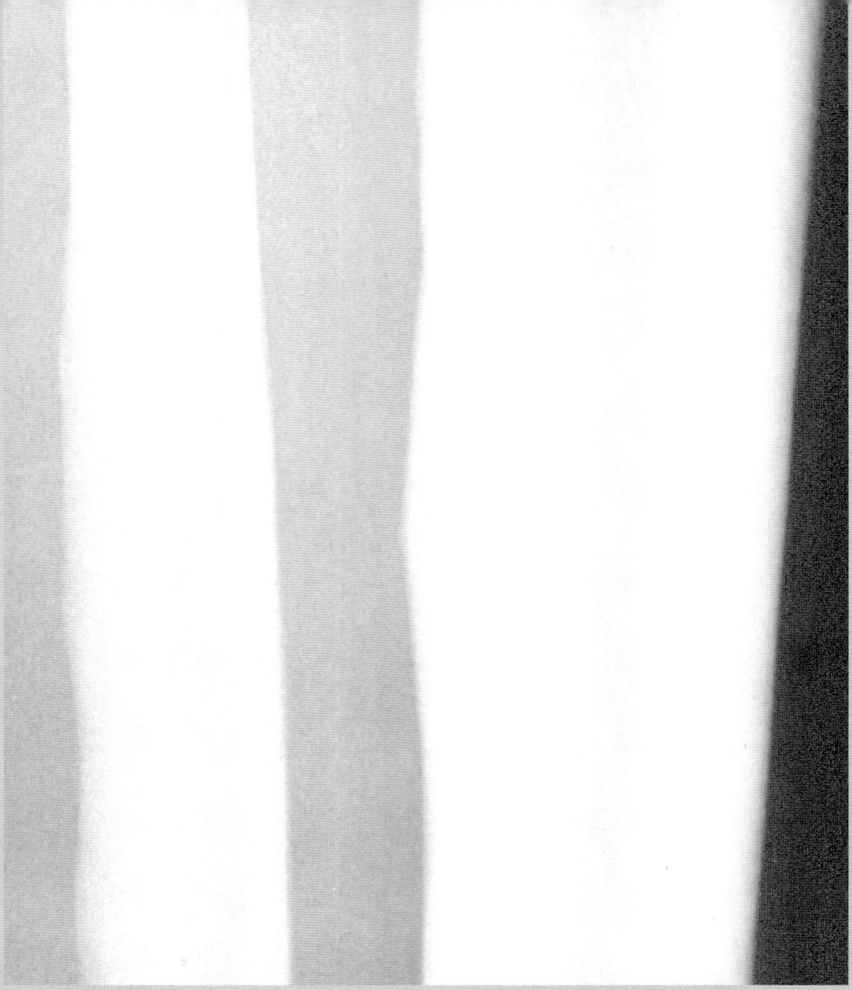

Figure 4.5 A stress fracture of the posteromedial aspect of the tibia (Detmer type I) is usually vertically orientated.

Figure 4.6 High-grade proximal left tibial stress fracture in the posteromedial cortex.

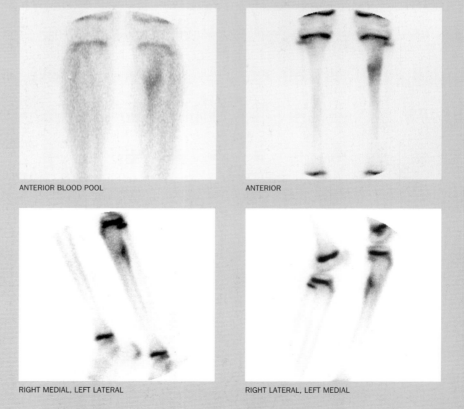

ANTERIOR BLOOD POOL

ANTERIOR

RIGHT MEDIAL, LEFT LATERAL

RIGHT LATERAL, LEFT MEDIAL

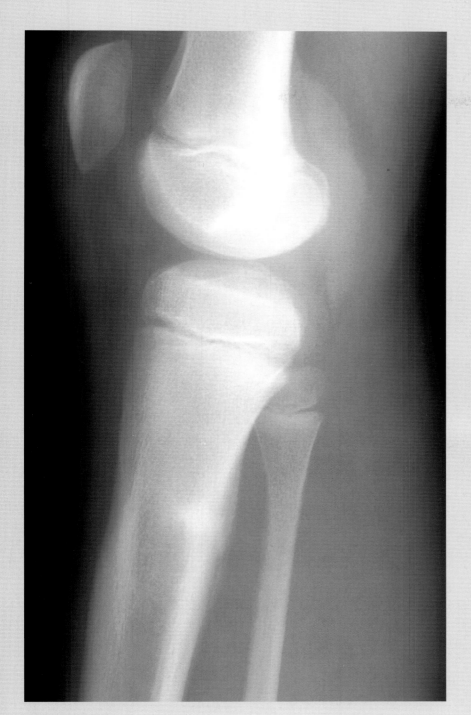

Figure 4.7 A common site of a stress fracture in the proximal tibia is posteriorly at a level just below that of the tibial tuberosity. This occurs often in adolescent athletes.

Figure 4.8 High-grade proximal left tibial full thickness stress fracture.

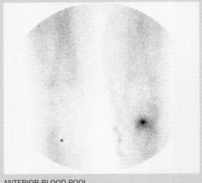

ANTERIOR BLOOD POOL

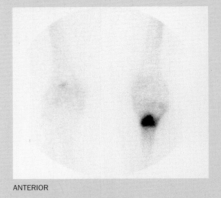

ANTERIOR

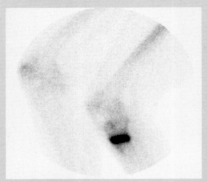

RIGHT MEDIAL, LEFT LATERAL

Figure 4.9 The commonest tibial stress fracture occurs beneath the medial tibial plateau. This stress fracture is not usually seen in athletes and is usually associated with decreased bone mineral. The stress fracture is shown on a bone scan. A plain film 1 week later shows a band of sclerosis (arrow).

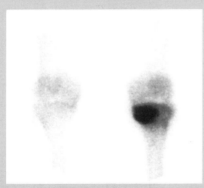

ANTERIOR

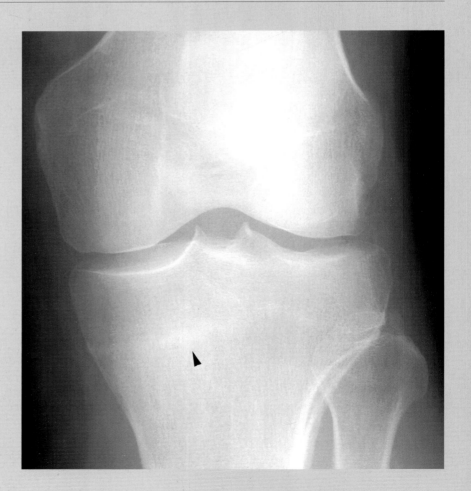

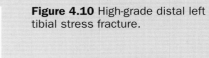

Figure 4.10 High-grade distal left tibial stress fracture.

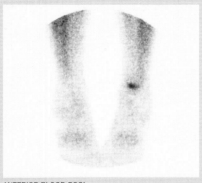

ANTERIOR BLOOD POOL

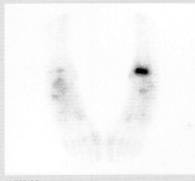

ANTERIOR

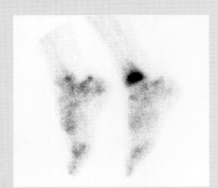

RIGHT MEDIAL, LEFT LATERAL

Figure 4.11 This distal metaphyseal stress fracture occurred after unaccustomed cross-country running.

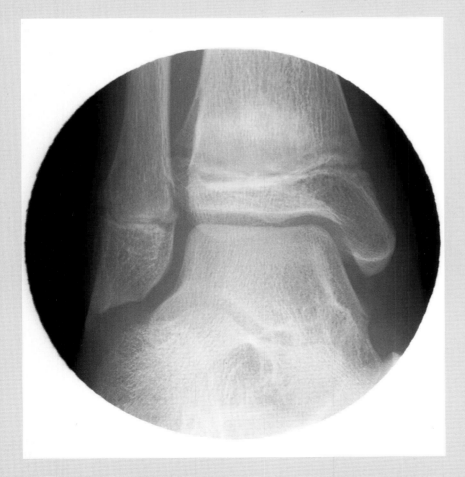

Figure 4.12 Left tibial stress fracture in the midshaft laterally—an uncommon site.

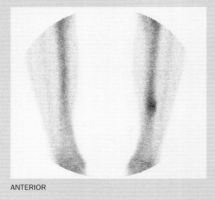

ANTERIOR

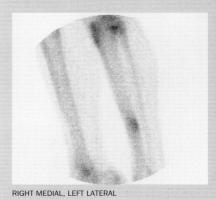

RIGHT MEDIAL, LEFT LATERAL

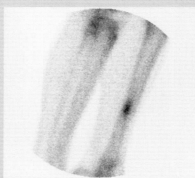

RIGHT LATERAL, LEFT MEDIAL

Figure 4.13 Very low-grade distal left fibular stress fracture involving the growth plate. Note the increased vascularity in the distal fibular physis on the blood pool image. Physeal fractures are frequently best detected on the blood pool images.

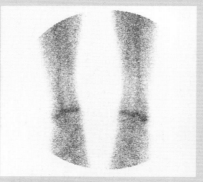

ANTERIOR BLOOD POOL

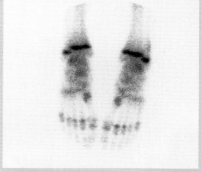

ANTERIOR

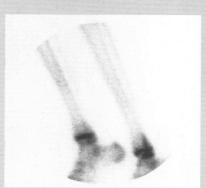

RIGHT MEDIAL, LEFT LATERAL

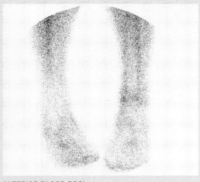

ANTERIOR BLOOD POOL

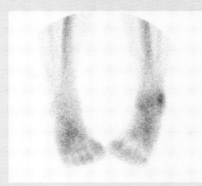

ANTERIOR

Figure 4.14 Distal left fibular stress fracture.

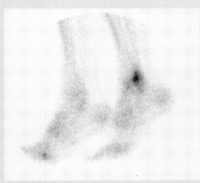

RIGHT MEDIAL, LEFT LATERAL

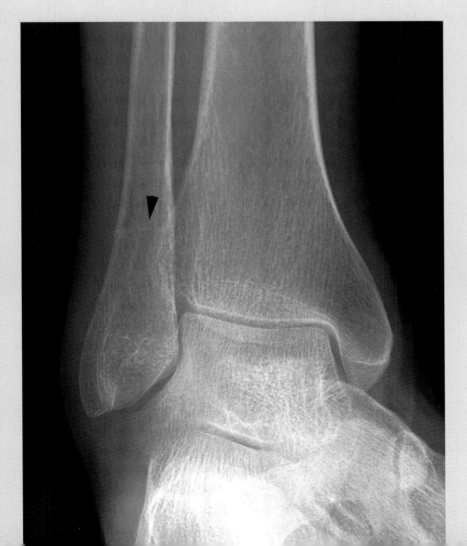

Figure 4.15 A stress fracture of the distal fibula is a common stress fracture and occurs just above the level of the distal tibiofibular joint. This fracture is confined almost always to recreational athletes or occasionally an elite athlete who is cross-training (e.g. a swimmer who takes up road running).

Figure 4.16 Bilateral distal fibular stress fractures. The fracture on the left is of higher grade as evidenced by the greater vascularity on the blood pool image and more intense uptake on the delayed images.

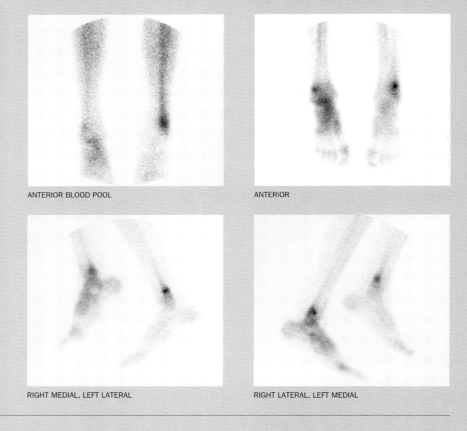

ANTERIOR BLOOD POOL

ANTERIOR

RIGHT MEDIAL, LEFT LATERAL

RIGHT LATERAL, LEFT MEDIAL

Figure 4.17 Stress fracture of the proximal shaft of the right fibula. There is mild diffuse stress reaction in the left fibular shaft.

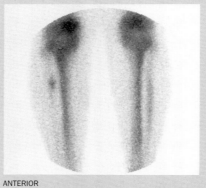

ANTERIOR

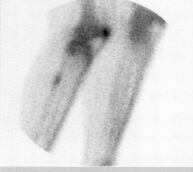

RIGHT LATERAL, LEFT MEDIAL

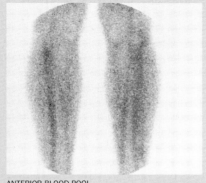

ANTERIOR BLOOD POOL

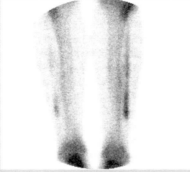

ANTERIOR

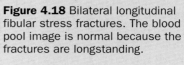

Figure 4.18 Bilateral longitudinal fibular stress fractures. The blood pool image is normal because the fractures are longstanding.

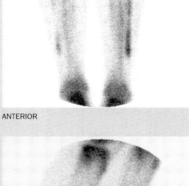

RIGHT MEDIAL, LEFT LATERAL

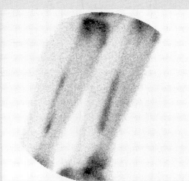

RIGHT LATERAL, LEFT MEDIAL

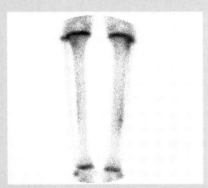

ANTERIOR

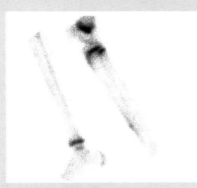

RIGHT MEDIAL, LEFT LATERAL

Figure 4.19 Low grade left anterior tibial shaft stress fracture. Anterior tibial shaft stress fractures are uncommon and are more prone to complications.

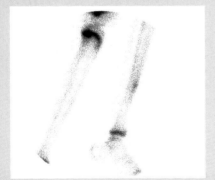

RIGHT LATERAL, LEFT MEDIAL

Figure 4.20 An anterior cortical stress fracture of the tibia is usually associated with jumping sports.

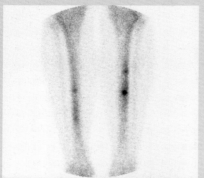

ANTERIOR

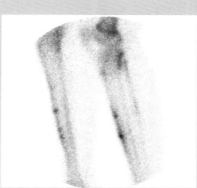

RIGHT MEDIAL, LEFT LATERAL

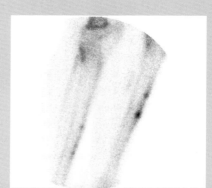

RIGHT LATERAL, LEFT MEDIAL

Figure 4.21 Multiple bilateral anterior tibial stress fractures.

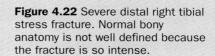

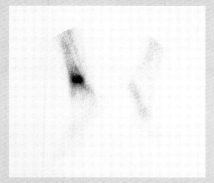

FROGLEG BLOOD POOL

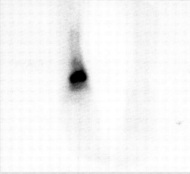

ANTERIOR

Figure 4.22 Severe distal right tibial stress fracture. Normal bony anatomy is not well defined because the fracture is so intense.

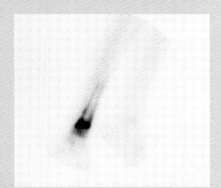

RIGHT LATERAL, LEFT MEDIAL

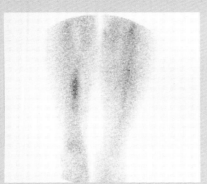

ANTERIOR BLOOD POOL

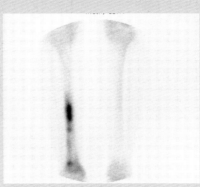

ANTERIOR

Figure 4.23 Linear stress fracture involving the right tibial midshaft with extension to the distal metaphysis. The higher grade portion of the fracture in the midshaft shows increased blood pool activity.

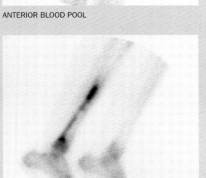

RIGHT LATERAL, LEFT MEDIAL

105

Figure 4.24 Linear stress fracture in the midshaft of the left tibia anteriorly.

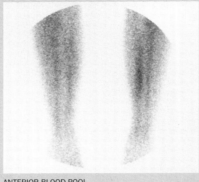

ANTERIOR BLOOD POOL

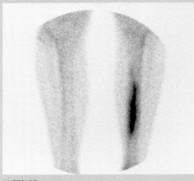

ANTERIOR

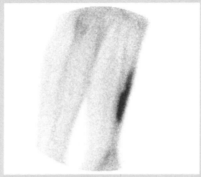

RIGHT LATERAL, LEFT MEDIAL

Figure 4.25 Spiral stress fracture of the distal right tibia, with the oblique component well demonstrated on the lateral view.

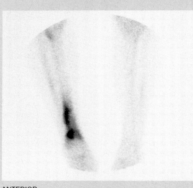

ANTERIOR

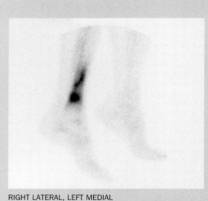

RIGHT LATERAL, LEFT MEDIAL

Figure 4.26 Stress fracture of the distal right tibia, with the majority of the fracture being transverse medially, but with a small spiral component extending superolaterally.

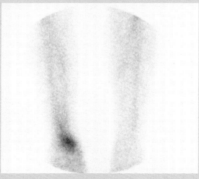

ANTERIOR BLOOD POOL

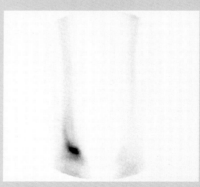

ANTERIOR

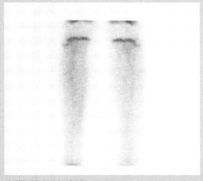

ANTERIOR BLOOD POOL

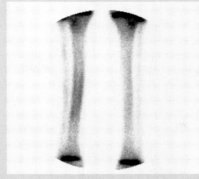

ANTERIOR

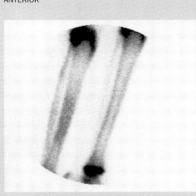

RIGHT MEDIAL, LEFT LATERAL

RIGHT LATERAL, LEFT MEDIAL

Figure 4.27 Plastic deformity fracture of the right tibia and fibula. Note the diffuse increase in uptake and bowing. This fracture was caused by heavy direct trauma to a 14-year-old during rugby football.

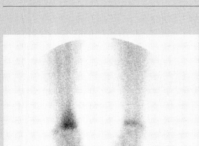

ANTERIOR BLOOD POOL

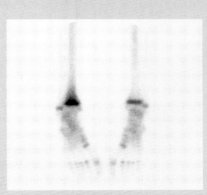

ANTERIOR

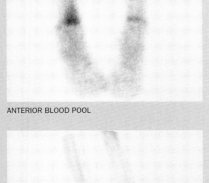

RIGHT MEDIAL, LEFT LATERAL

Figure 4.28 Stress fracture in the distal left tibial growth plate with activity flaring into the metaphysis. Care must be taken to exclude osteomyelitis which can have a similar appearance in the young.

Figure 4.29 Paget's disease of the right tibia. As with all nuclear medicine, the clinical context is very important. This scan appearance could be seen with fracture, but in this instance was due to Paget's disease.

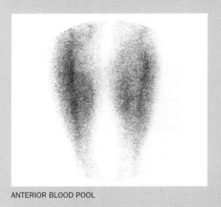

ANTERIOR BLOOD POOL

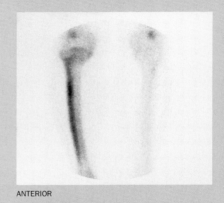

ANTERIOR

Periosteal reaction (Figs 4.30–4.33)

Periosteal reaction was demonstrated by Detmer in the more acute cases of type II shin pain. This is the condition commonly referred to in nuclear medicine practice as 'shin splints'. As previously discussed, because of confusion surrounding the term, it is probably best avoided. The linear increase in uptake in a periosteal distribution is best described as periosteal reaction, as this agrees with the clinical appearance, bone scan findings and histology.

Periosteal reaction occurs in runners and participants in any sport involving running. It is frequently associated with minor foot biomechanical abnormalities such as abnormal pronation, which causes excessive repetitive stress at muscle origin sites in the tibia (Sharpey's fibres). Periosteal new bone on X-ray is an uncommon finding and usually denotes chronicity. The same process may occur in the fibula.

Bone-scan appearance

Characteristically, in periosteal reaction there is no increase in vascularity in the early views. While there is some disagreement and controversy in this area, our view is that the lack of abnormal vascularity on the early views is the typical appearance in periosteal reaction. Focal areas of increased vascularity favour superimposed stress fracture.

The delayed bone-scan images show a linear band of increased uptake of isotope along the posteromedial border of the tibia. Much less commonly, the fibula may be involved. It is important to note that in some cases the tibial uptake may be very irregular, with areas of greater uptake along the linear band. Clinically these areas are often 'lumpy' and tender to palpation and probably represent areas of greater traction injury. Occasionally differentiation of coexisting stress fracture can be difficult.

There is debate as to whether there is a continuum between periosteal reaction and stress fracture. While the two entities may coexist, we do not support the theory of a continuum. Most stress fractures occur with no evidence of associated periosteal reaction and in the majority of cases periosteal reaction is seen without fracture.

It must be remembered that more chronic periosteal disengagement may show no abnormality on a bone scan. The frequency of this has not been well documented to date.

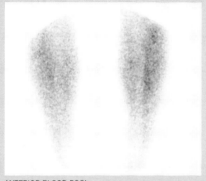

ANTERIOR BLOOD POOL

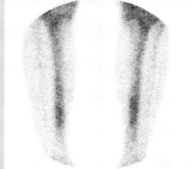
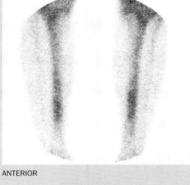

ANTERIOR

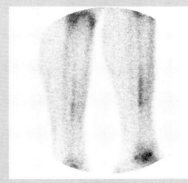

RIGHT MEDIAL, LEFT LATERAL

RIGHT LATERAL, LEFT MEDIAL

Figure 4.30 Typical periosteal reaction with linear increase in uptake in the posteromedial border of the mid tibiae seen best in the medial views. Note that there is no bony hypervascularity in the early view.

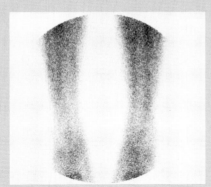

ANTERIOR BLOOD POOL

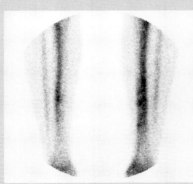

ANTERIOR

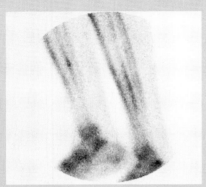

RIGHT MEDIAL, LEFT LATERAL

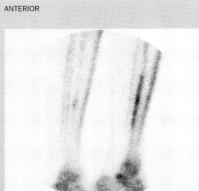

RIGHT LATERAL, LEFT MEDIAL

Figure 4.31 More severe posteromedial periosteal reaction in the left tibia. The right tibia also shows mild periosteal uptake with a small focal area of greater activity, but no abnormality on the blood pool image.

Figure 4.32 Bilateral periosteal reaction. Irregular linear increase in uptake in the posteromedial borders of the tibiae, but with focal areas of greater uptake. The absence of focal increase in vascularity on the blood pool image helps differentiate periosteal reaction from stress fractures in the acute phase.

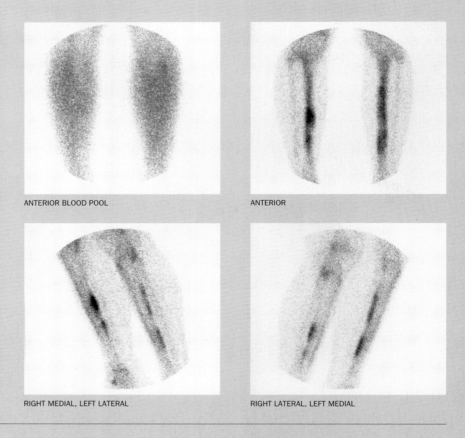

ANTERIOR BLOOD POOL

ANTERIOR

RIGHT MEDIAL, LEFT LATERAL

RIGHT LATERAL, LEFT MEDIAL

Figure 4.33 Bilateral midtibial posteromedial periosteal reaction demonstrating the most common appearance of uniform periosteal increase in uptake. The normal blood pool views (not shown) in this case were evidence against linear fracture.

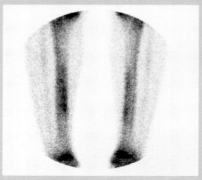

ANTERIOR

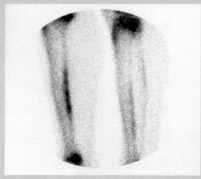

RIGHT MEDIAL, LEFT LATERAL

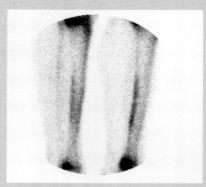

RIGHT LATERAL, LEFT MEDIAL

It is important to have a feel for the normal appearance of the bone scan in athletes. Any asymptomatic runner may show some degree of prominence of the borders of the tibiae, particularly a mild diffuse increase in anterior tibial uptake. This should not be over-interpreted as pathology. Only in the more extreme cases of diffuse anterior tibial uptake should a pathological process be considered (Figs 4.34 and 4.35).

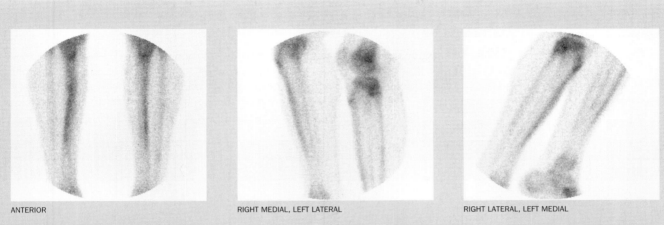

ANTERIOR   RIGHT MEDIAL, LEFT LATERAL   RIGHT LATERAL, LEFT MEDIAL

Figure 4.34 Normal appearance of the tibiae in a runner, showing prominent uptake anteriorly due to diffuse anterior stress remodelling.

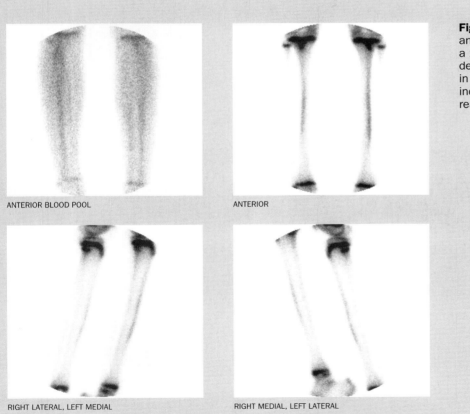

ANTERIOR BLOOD POOL   ANTERIOR

RIGHT LATERAL, LEFT MEDIAL   RIGHT MEDIAL, LEFT LATERAL

Figure 4.35 Prominent diffuse anterolateral tibial stress reaction in a 15-year-old high jumper. This degree of uptake is beyond the norm in athletic young patients and indicates a pathological stress reaction.

Compartment syndromes

The compartment syndromes (Detmer type III injuries) show no abnormality on the isotope bone scan. Studies have been published utilising the washout of isotopes, particularly thallium-201, on both planar and SPECT imaging. The technique has not lived up to its initial hopes and currently there is no widely accepted nuclear medicine procedure to diagnose this condition.

Other causes (Figs 4.36–4.38)

As previously discussed, there are many causes of exercise-induced leg pain and, as with all syndromes in sports medicine, it must be remembered that some of these conditions may coexist. In any one patient there may be evidence of both periosteal reaction and stress fracture. Conversely the presence of periosteal reaction does not exclude a compartment syndrome being the primary cause of symptoms.

Figure 4.36 Peritibial vascularity with no bony abnormality on the delayed views. This degree of peritibial vascularity is unusual and is probably pathological; however, the exact pathophysiology is unknown. The normal delayed images exclude acute periosteal reaction and stress fracture.

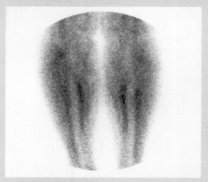
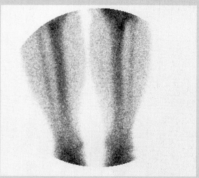

ANTERIOR BLOOD POOL   ANTERIOR

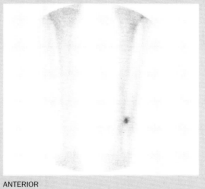

ANTERIOR   RIGHT MEDIAL, LEFT LATERAL

Figure 4.37 Calcification in the tibiofibular interosseous ligament following trauma. Plain X-ray may be normal early in this process, but later will demonstrate calcification.

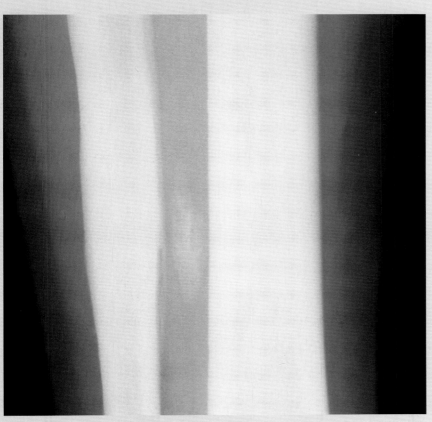

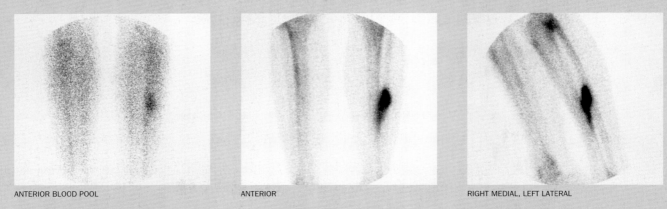

ANTERIOR BLOOD POOL ANTERIOR RIGHT MEDIAL, LEFT LATERAL

Figure 4.38 Fracture through old calcification bridging the tibiofibular interosseous ligament following recent trauma. The X-ray showed mature calcification secondary to a previous injury 20 years before. Recent direct trauma to the site resulted in fracture through the calcification.

Bibliography

Andrish, J, Bergfield, M, Walheim, J, A prospective study on the management of shin splints, *J Bone & J Surg* [Am] 56: 1974, pp 1697–700

Batt, ME, Shin splints: a review of terminology, *Clin J Sport* 5: 1995, pp 53–7

Batt, ME, Ugalde, V, Anderson, MW, Shelton, DK, A prospective controlled study of diagnostic imaging for acute shin splints, *Medicine & Science in Sport & Exercise* 30: 1998, pp 1564–71

Blank, S, Transverse tibial stress fractures: a special problem, *Am J Sports Med* 9: 1981, pp 322–5

Detmer, DE, Chronic shin splints. Classification & management of medial tibial stress syndrome, *Sports Med* 3: 1986, pp 436–46

Harcke, HT, Mandell, GA, Scintigraphic evaluation of the growth plate, *Sem Nuc Med* 23: 1993, pp 266–73

Holder, LE, Michael, RH, The specific scintigraphic pattern of shin splints in the lower leg. Concise communication, *J Nucl Med* 25: 1984, pp 865–9

Michael, RH, Holder, LE, The Soleus syndrome. A cause of medial tibial stress (shin splints), *Am J Sports Med* 13: 1985, pp 87–94

Milgrove, C, Chism, R, Geladi, M, et al., Negative bone scans in impending tibial stress fractures: a report of 3 cases, *Am J Sports Med* 12: 1984, pp 488–91

Mills, GQ, Marymont, JH, Murphy, DA, Bone scan utilisation in the differential diagnosis of exercise-induced lower extremity pain, *Clinical Orthopaedics & Related Research* 149: 1980, pp 207–10

Mubarak, SJ, Gould, RN, Forlee, Y, Schmidt, D, Hargens, A, The medial tibial stress syndrome: A cause of shin splints, *Am J Sports Med* 10: 1982, pp 201–5

Rettig, AC, Shelbourne, KD, McCarroll, JR, Bisesi, M, Watts, J, The natural history & treatment of delayed union stress fractures of the anterior cortex of the tibia, *Am J Sports Med* 16: 1988, pp 250–5

Zwas, ST, Elankovich, L, Frank, G, Interpretation and classification of bone scintigraphic findings in stress fractures, *J Nucl Med* 28: 1987, pp 452–7

5 The knee

Acute knee injuries occur frequently in sport and are usually the result of direct trauma, a twisting injury, or a combination of both. These injuries are particularly prevalent in contact sports, with the vulnerable anatomical position of the knee being a contributing factor. Chronic conditions are also common in both recreational and elite athletes, often as a result of overuse.

Following acute knee injuries, the role of the bone scan is largely confined to the diagnosis of occult fractures. With chronic knee pain the role of bone scan is more diverse and is useful in identifying bone stress, stress fractures, degenerative change, osteonecrosis, enthesopathies and occasionally soft tissue problems. Injuries to menisci, the cruciate ligaments and collateral ligaments are best demonstrated using MRI.

Tips on technique

The views obtained with the bone scan of the knees are the anterior, lateral, medial and posterior views. The joints above and below the knee should be included in the examination so the images will cover the lower limb from the pelvis to the feet (Fig. 5.1).

In particular cases, special views may aid in the diagnosis. For example, an intercondylar view is helpful in the evaluation of osteochondritis dissecans. This is performed with the knee partially flexed to approximately 25 degrees and the camera positioned perpendicular to the tibial plateau. Using this view, the area of involvement is seen without overlap, confirming the characteristic site and uptake of this process.

If patellar fracture is suspected in younger patients, a similar view may help image the patella without the underlying distal femoral growth plate activity obscuring the fracture. The optimal degree of camera tilt, either caudal or cranial, needs to be tailored to the individual.

SPECT views of the knees have been advocated by some authors.

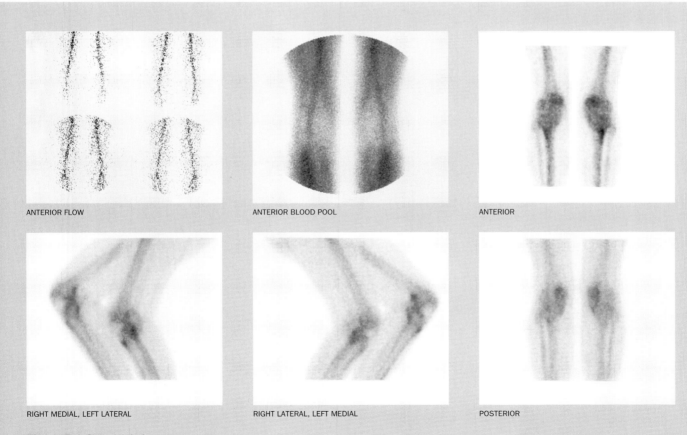

ANTERIOR FLOW

ANTERIOR BLOOD POOL

ANTERIOR

RIGHT MEDIAL, LEFT LATERAL

RIGHT LATERAL, LEFT MEDIAL

POSTERIOR

Figure 5.1 Standard views.

Fractures (Figs 5.2–5.22)

Fractures, whether occult or resulting from chronic bone stress, exhibit a characteristic increase in blood flow, blood pool and delayed focal increase in uptake.

Commonly a bone scan is necessary to diagnose osteochondral fractures as these fractures can be extremely difficult to see on plain film. The presence of an osteochondral fracture should be suspected when knee pain persists after trauma. It is also important to remember that a fracture in the subchondral bone may be covered by normal cartilage and an arthroscopy can be perfectly normal. This is because cartilage is more resilient than the underlying bone. Even if the cartilage is damaged, a cartilaginous flap may be difficult to identify at arthroscopy.

The bone scan also plays a useful role in the immature athlete. Acute and stress injury occur at growth plates and these changes may be difficult to see on the initial plain films due to normal inherent irregularity. On the delayed images it may be difficult to be confident of the diagnosis of subtle growth plate disruption, due to the high degree of physeal activity. The changes are often better seen on the blood pool image, where the difference in uptake is greater.

Figure 5.2 Small osteochondral fracture of the left medial femoral condyle. Subtle uptake is seen on both the early and delayed views on the inferior articular surface, indicating a low-grade fracture.

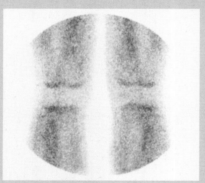
ANTERIOR BLOOD POOL

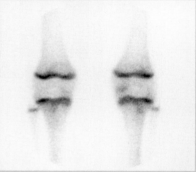
ANTERIOR

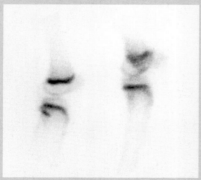
RIGHT LATERAL, LEFT MEDIAL

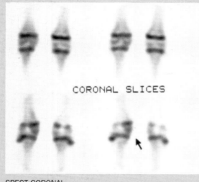

CORONAL SLICES

SPECT CORONAL

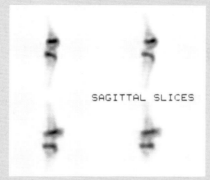

SAGITTAL SLICES

SPECT SAGITTAL

Figure 5.3 Low-grade osteochondral fracture of the right medial femoral condyle posteriorly seen on SPECT images. The planar images showed activity similar to that seen in Fig. 5.2. In the authors' experience, adequate localisation can usually be achieved in the knee with multiple planar images.

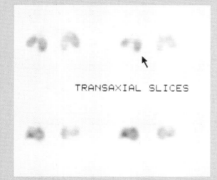

TRANSAXIAL SLICES

SPECT TRANSAXIAL

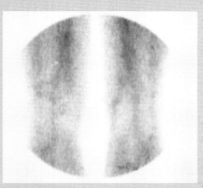

ANTERIOR BLOOD POOL

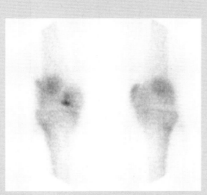

ANTERIOR

Figure 5.4 Small osteochondral fracture of the right medial femoral condyle involving the patello-femoral articular surface. Direct patellar trauma is a common mechanism for this type of fracture.

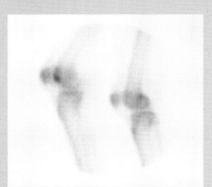

RIGHT MEDIAL, LEFT LATERAL

Figure 5.5 Moderate osteochondral fracture of the right lateral femoral condyle. The maximal activity is at the joint surface, but the increase in uptake extends into the condyle. On the left side, the increase in uptake over the medial edge of the medial femoral condyle is outside the articular surface and is due to medial ligament injury.

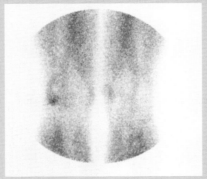 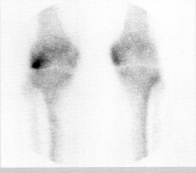

ANTERIOR BLOOD POOL

ANTERIOR

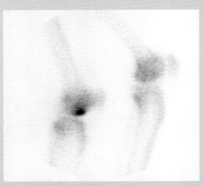

RIGHT LATERAL, LEFT MEDIAL

Figure 5.6 A subtle subchondral fracture of the medial femoral condyle.

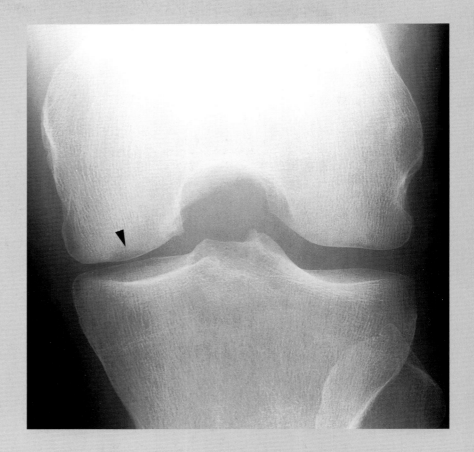

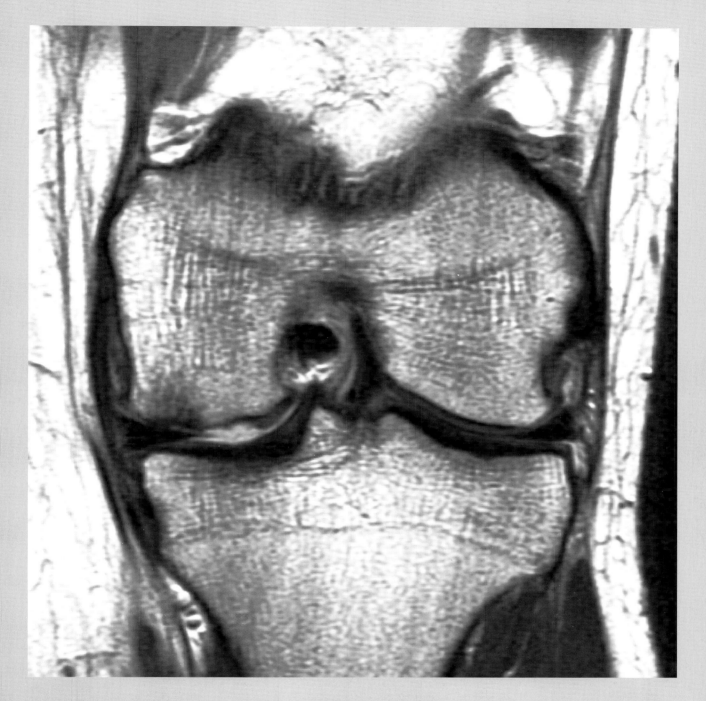

Figure 5.7 This coronal MR image shows a chondral defect with subchondral bony changes.

Figure 5.8 Bilateral osteochondral fractures in the medial femoral condyles.

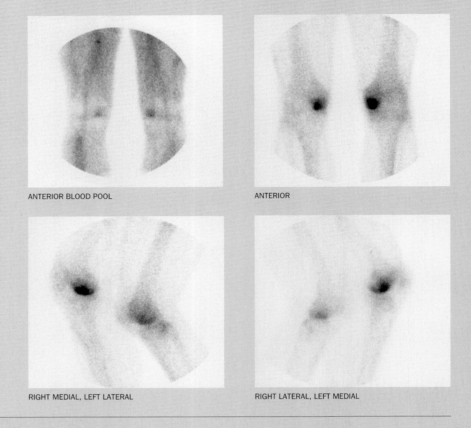

ANTERIOR BLOOD POOL

ANTERIOR

RIGHT MEDIAL, LEFT LATERAL

RIGHT LATERAL, LEFT MEDIAL

Figure 5.9 Osteochondral fracture of the posterior aspect of the left lateral femoral condyle. The uptake is in the articular surface.

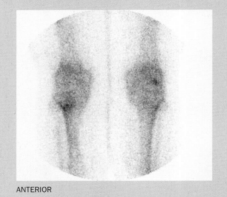

ANTERIOR

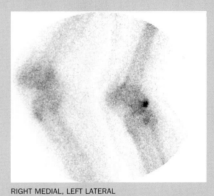

RIGHT MEDIAL, LEFT LATERAL

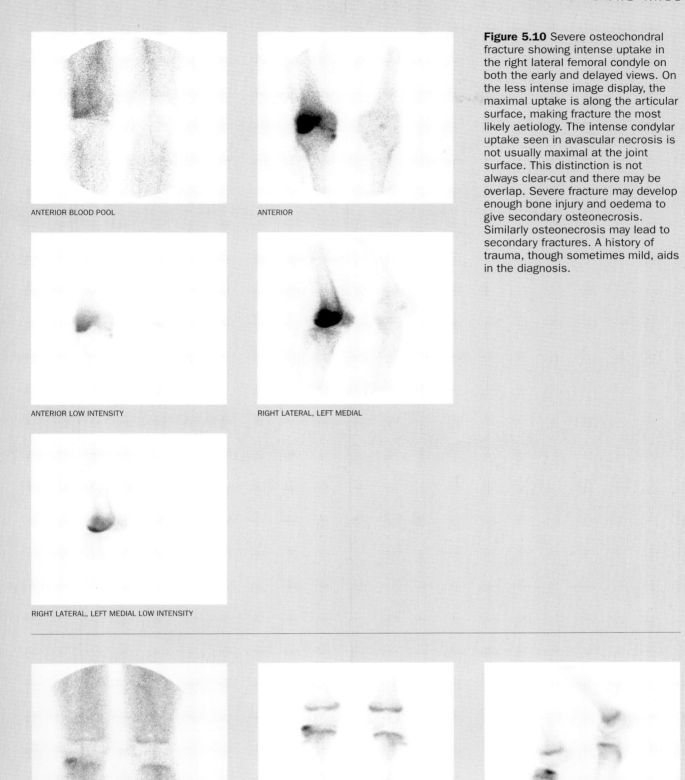

ANTERIOR BLOOD POOL

ANTERIOR

ANTERIOR LOW INTENSITY

RIGHT LATERAL, LEFT MEDIAL

RIGHT LATERAL, LEFT MEDIAL LOW INTENSITY

Figure 5.10 Severe osteochondral fracture showing intense uptake in the right lateral femoral condyle on both the early and delayed views. On the less intense image display, the maximal uptake is along the articular surface, making fracture the most likely aetiology. The intense condylar uptake seen in avascular necrosis is not usually maximal at the joint surface. This distinction is not always clear-cut and there may be overlap. Severe fracture may develop enough bone injury and oedema to give secondary osteonecrosis. Similarly osteonecrosis may lead to secondary fractures. A history of trauma, though sometimes mild, aids in the diagnosis.

ANTERIOR BLOOD POOL

ANTERIOR

RIGHT LATERAL, LEFT MEDIAL

Figure 5.11 Small osteochondral fracture of the right lateral tibial plateau. The typical localised horizontal linear blood pool and delayed uptake are separate from the growth plate activity and are confined to one side of the joint.

Figure 5.12 Bilateral medial tibial plateau fractures. This type of fracture is more commonly seen as an insufficiency fracture in the osteoporotic patient.

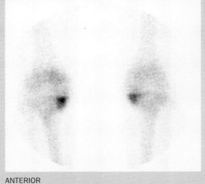

ANTERIOR

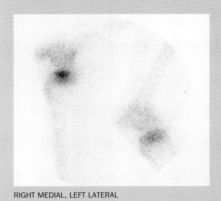

RIGHT MEDIAL, LEFT LATERAL

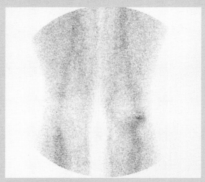

RIGHT LATERAL, LEFT MEDIAL

Figure 5.13 Left lateral tibial plateau compression fracture at the articular surface with activity flaring into the subarticular bone.

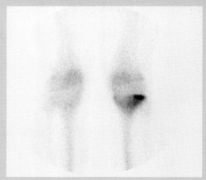

ANTERIOR BLOOD POOL

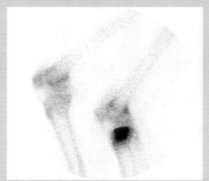

ANTERIOR

RIGHT MEDIAL, LEFT LATERAL

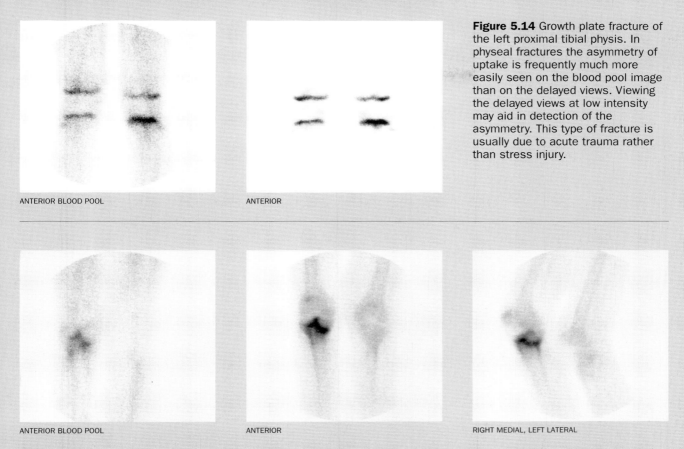

Figure 5.14 Growth plate fracture of the left proximal tibial physis. In physeal fractures the asymmetry of uptake is frequently much more easily seen on the blood pool image than on the delayed views. Viewing the delayed views at low intensity may aid in detection of the asymmetry. This type of fracture is usually due to acute trauma rather than stress injury.

ANTERIOR BLOOD POOL

ANTERIOR

ANTERIOR BLOOD POOL

ANTERIOR

RIGHT MEDIAL, LEFT LATERAL

Figure 5.15 Comminuted fracture of the proximal right tibia. This fracture is due to acute trauma rather than stress injury. Despite the severity of the fracture, the X-ray was normal.

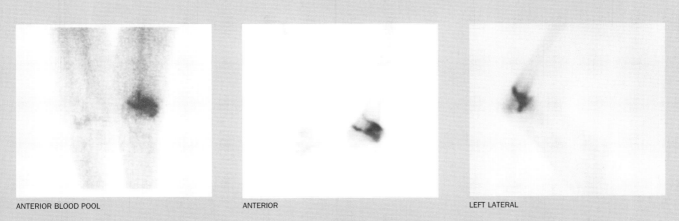

ANTERIOR BLOOD POOL

ANTERIOR

LEFT LATERAL

Figure 5.16 Comminuted fracture of the distal left femur. While primarily intercondylar, part of the fracture extends to involve the joint. This is an insufficiency fracture.

Figure 5.17 Avulsion fracture at the superolateral aspect of the left patella. The left knee was the symptomatic knee. Note the small osteochondral fracture in the right medial femoral condyle.

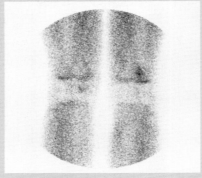

ANTERIOR BLOOD POOL

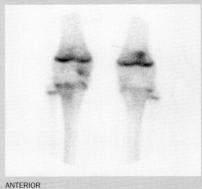

ANTERIOR

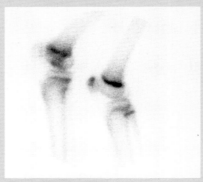

RIGHT MEDIAL, LEFT LATERAL

Figure 5.18 Avulsion fracture at the upper pole of the right patella. The early view (not included) showed focal hyperaemia at the upper pole. The focal hyperaemia in conjunction with the history of recent trauma is important in distinguishing this condition from an enthesopathy.

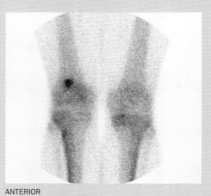

ANTERIOR

RIGHT LATERAL, LEFT MEDIAL

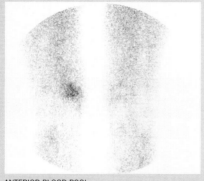

ANTERIOR BLOOD POOL

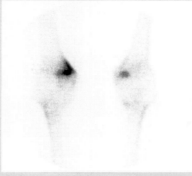

ANTERIOR

Figure 5.19 Bilateral distal femoral stress fractures. The left fracture was asymptomatic—a common clinical occurrence because the pain of the more severe injury prevents further exercise on the left leg.

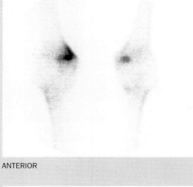

RIGHT MEDIAL, LEFT LATERAL

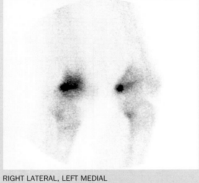

RIGHT LATERAL, LEFT MEDIAL

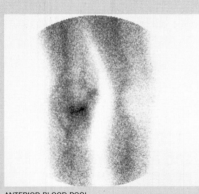

ANTERIOR BLOOD POOL

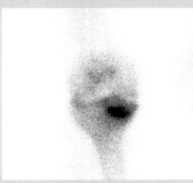

ANTERIOR ZOOM

Figure 5.20 Stress fracture of the right medial tibial condyle, not involving the articular surface. This is a common site for a stress fracture.

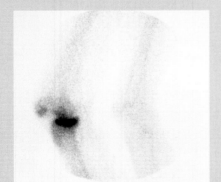

RIGHT MEDIAL, LEFT LATERAL

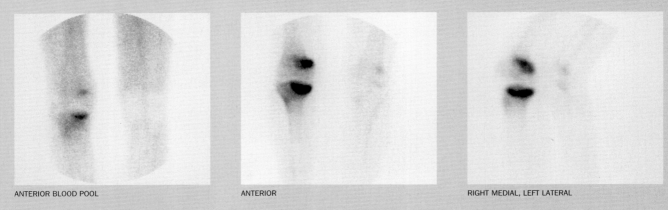

ANTERIOR BLOOD POOL   ANTERIOR   RIGHT MEDIAL, LEFT LATERAL

Figure 5.21 Stress fractures in the right medial tibial and distal femoral condyles.

Figure 5.22 Stress fracture in the distal left femur related to a knee prosthesis. This occurred in the absence of acute trauma.

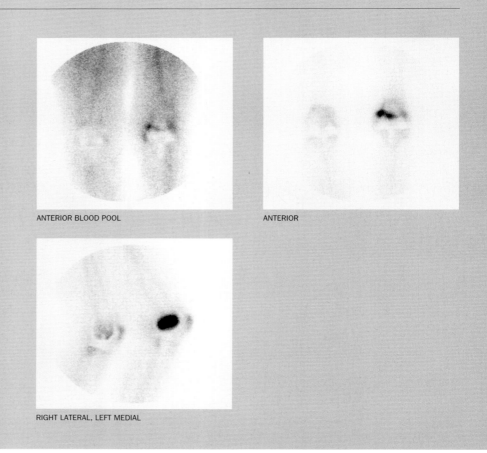

ANTERIOR BLOOD POOL   ANTERIOR

RIGHT LATERAL, LEFT MEDIAL

Synovitis and degenerative changes (Figs 5.23–5.27)

The bone scan is helpful in distinguishing synovitis and degenerative change from fracture. It can also demonstrate the site of activity of arthritis, showing either diffusely increased or focal uptake in the articular surfaces. It is not as good at determining the aetiology of the arthritis.

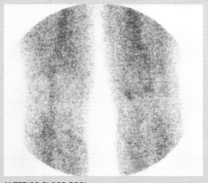

ANTERIOR BLOOD POOL

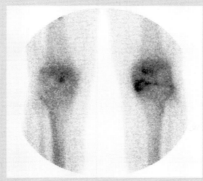

ANTERIOR

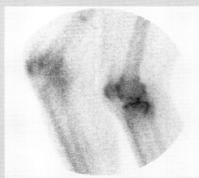

RIGHT LATERAL, LEFT MEDIAL

RIGHT MEDIAL, LEFT LATERAL

Figure 5.23 Arthritis in the left knee. There is increased uptake of isotope in the articular surfaces of all compartments of the left knee and, to a lesser extent, in the patello-femoral compartment of the right knee.

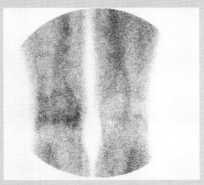

ANTERIOR BLOOD POOL

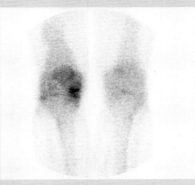

ANTERIOR

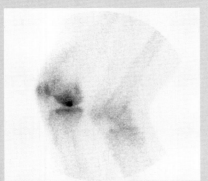

RIGHT MEDIAL, LEFT LATERAL

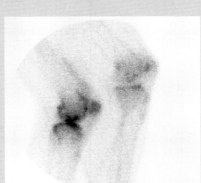

RIGHT LATERAL, LEFT MEDIAL

Figure 5.24 Arthritis in both knees, more marked on the right. There is increased uptake in the articular surfaces of both knees and in the suprapatellar bursa of the right knee. Note that it is difficult to localise the exact site of uptake on the anterior or posterior views, but the lateral and medial views are very helpful.

Figure 5.25 Arthritis in the right knee with marked soft tissue uptake in the suprapatellar bursa, usually indicating the presence of a joint effusion.

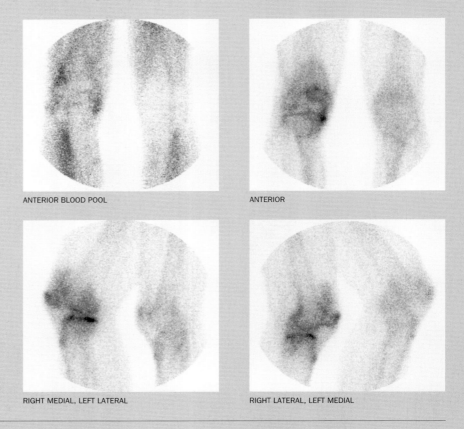

ANTERIOR BLOOD POOL

ANTERIOR

RIGHT MEDIAL, LEFT LATERAL

RIGHT LATERAL, LEFT MEDIAL

Figure 5.26 Right Baker's cyst and left suprapatellar bursa effusion. The blood pool image demonstrates hyperaemia in both knees, indicating synovitis, though with only mild uptake on the delayed images. Low-grade soft tissue activity is seen posterior to the right knee on the medial view, indicating a Baker's cyst.

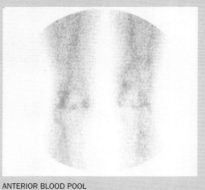

ANTERIOR BLOOD POOL

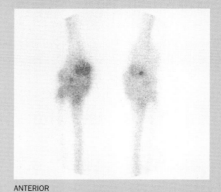

ANTERIOR

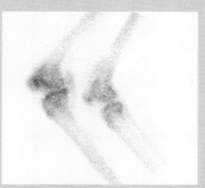

RIGHT MEDIAL, LEFT LATERAL

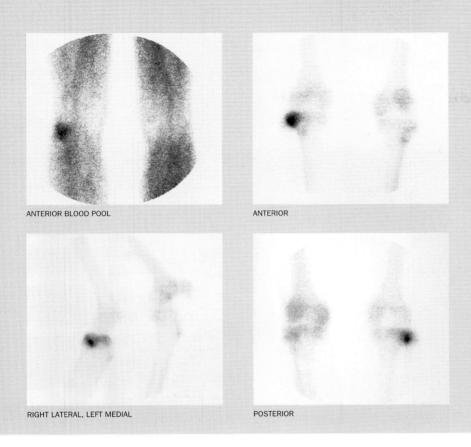

ANTERIOR BLOOD POOL

ANTERIOR

RIGHT LATERAL, LEFT MEDIAL

POSTERIOR

Figure 5.27 Traumatic synovitis in the right proximal tibiofibular joint. It is important to image the entire fibula, including the distal tibiofibular joint, to detect distal syndesmosis and interosseous membrane injuries.

Osteonecrosis (Figs 5.28 and 5.29)

Bone scans are sensitive and useful in the detection of osteonecrosis. This painful process usually involves subchondral bone and may be quite extensive, with little evidence seen on plain films. The scan shows localised intense increase in blood flow, blood pool and delayed bone uptake in the femoral condyles. Some experts assert that a similar appearance on the tibial side of the joint is due to fracture. In fact, the aetiology of osteonecrosis is uncertain and in some cases may be secondary to fracture.

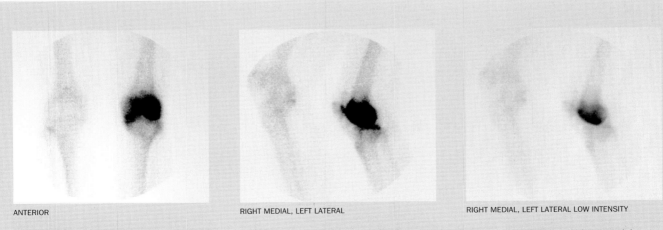

ANTERIOR

RIGHT MEDIAL, LEFT LATERAL

RIGHT MEDIAL, LEFT LATERAL LOW INTENSITY

Figure 5.28 Osteonecrosis of the condyles of the left femur, more marked laterally. Fracture with very extensive condylar involvement can have the same appearance.

Figure 5.29 Subchondral demineralisation and compression due to osteonecrosis.

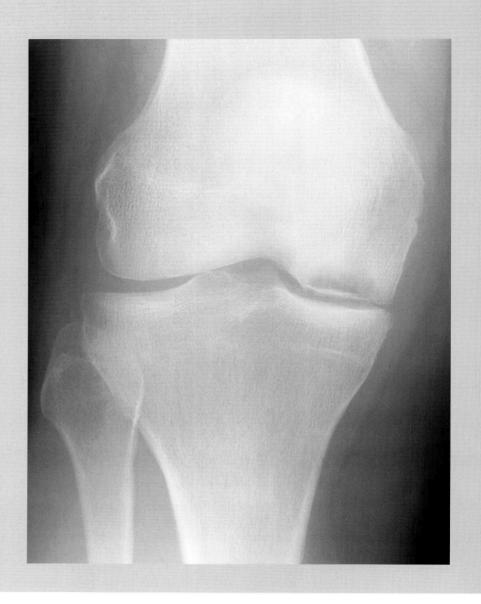

Enthesopathies (Figs 5.30–5.37)

Chronic knee pain can result from enthesopathy at tendon or ligament insertion sites. Common enthesopathies are related to the superior and inferior poles of the patella, the tibial tuberosity, gastrocnemius insertions, the insertion of the collateral ligaments and the ilio-tibial band insertion. On the bone scan the early views are frequently normal, while the delayed views show a small focus of uptake localised to the insertion site. If there is a significant increase in vascularity in the region on the early views, then associated tendonitis is likely.

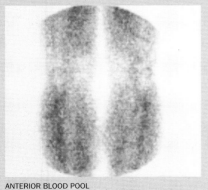

ANTERIOR BLOOD POOL

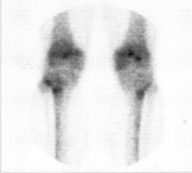

ANTERIOR

Figure 5.30 Bilateral enthesopathies at the lower poles of both patellae (jumper's knees) and in both tibial tubercles. Note that the blood pool images are usually normal in this condition.

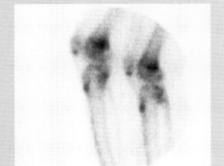

RIGHT MEDIAL, LEFT LATERAL

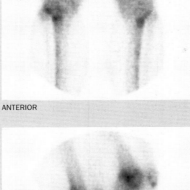

RIGHT LATERAL, LEFT MEDIAL

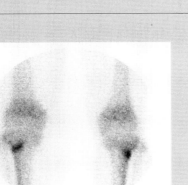

ANTERIOR

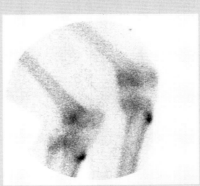

RIGHT LATERAL, LEFT MEDIAL

Figure 5.31 Bilateral tibial tubercle enthesopathies at the insertion of the patellar ligaments.

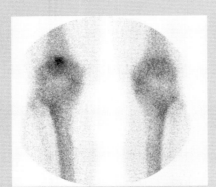

ANTERIOR

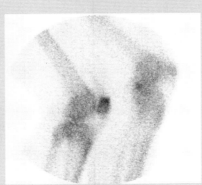

RIGHT LATERAL, LEFT MEDIAL

Figure 5.32 Enthesopathy at the upper pole of the right patella at the quadriceps insertion. Note that the activity is maximal at the anterior edge of the upper pole, distinguishing enthesopathy from focal retropatellar arthritis.

Figure 5.33 Patellar tendinopathy with associated enthesopathy at the inferior pole of the patella.

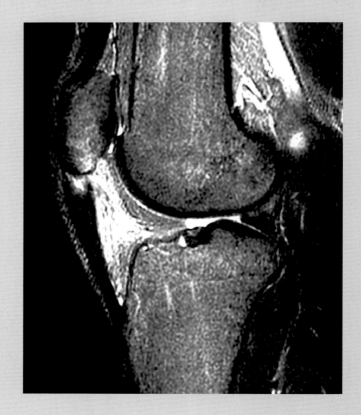

Figure 5.34 Soft tissue contusion adjacent to the quadriceps insertion at the lateral edge of the left patella. The blood pool image shows hyperaemia at this site, with only minor bony reaction.

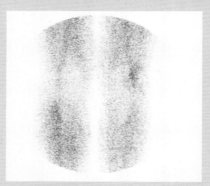

ANTERIOR BLOOD POOL

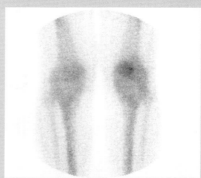

ANTERIOR

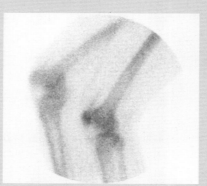

RIGHT MEDIAL, LEFT LATERAL

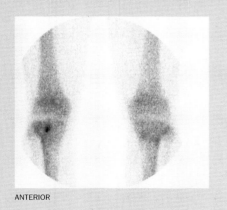
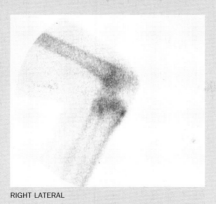

ANTERIOR · RIGHT LATERAL

Figure 5.35 Enthesopathy at the insertion of the right ilio-tibial band. This is much less common than patellar enthesopathies in the authors' experience.

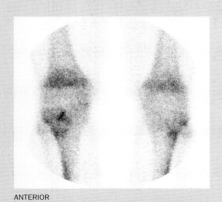
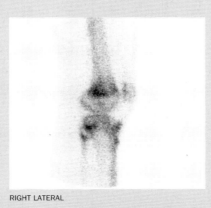

ANTERIOR · RIGHT LATERAL

Figure 5.36 Calcification at the insertion of the right ilio-tibial band. Note that the increase in uptake extends anteriorly from the insertion site on the lateral view.

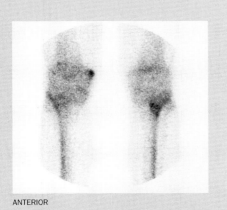
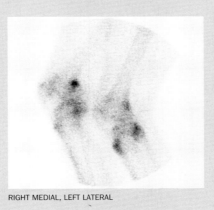

ANTERIOR · RIGHT MEDIAL, LEFT LATERAL

Figure 5.37 Enthesopathy at the posterosuperior edge of the right medial femoral condyle. It is difficult to distinguish between the insertions of the quadriceps and the medial head of the gastrocnemius. Note that the focus of uptake lies above the joint surface posteriorly. It is posterosuperior to the medial ligament insertion site.

Ligaments (Figs 5.38–5.40)

Although ligament injuries are best imaged using ultrasound or MRI, knowledge of the bone scan appearance of these is essential in the interpretation of bone scans of the knees. Lateral and medial collateral ligament injuries are the most commonly seen ligament injuries in nuclear medicine. Cruciate ligament injuries rarely present to nuclear medicine other than to exclude associated subchondral fracture. With cruciate ligament injury, if the tear involves the bone/ligament interface, there will be focal increased uptake on bone scan, otherwise the scan may show only diffuse traumatic synovitis in the acute phase.

Figure 5.38 Medial ligament avulsion injury in the left knee. The early view indicates the extent of soft tissue injury in the line of the medial ligament. The delayed image shows uptake at the insertion site.

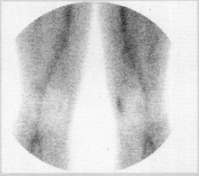

ANTERIOR BLOOD POOL

ANTERIOR

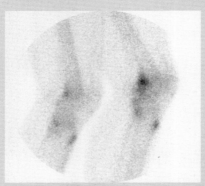

RIGHT LATERAL, LEFT MEDIAL

Figure 5.39 Right medial ligament injury. The blood pool image demonstrates the linear vascularity along the ligament, with increased delayed uptake at the site of the traction injury on the femoral insertion.

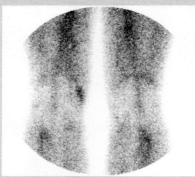

ANTERIOR BLOOD POOL

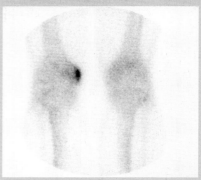

ANTERIOR

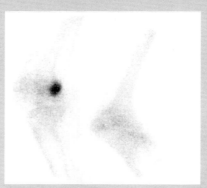

RIGHT MEDIAL, LEFT LATERAL

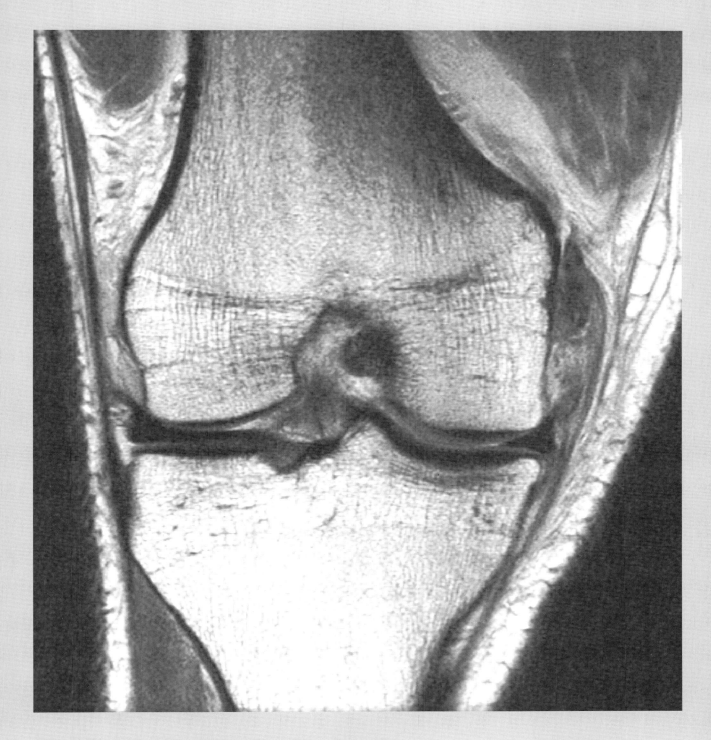

Figure 5.40 Proximal medial collateral ligament injury shown by MRI.

Osteochondritis dissecans (Figs 5.41 and 5.42)

The typical appearance is a small focus of increased isotope uptake in the lateral side of the medial femoral condyle. The scan can help diagnose the condition. The degree of uptake can also help assess the degree of healing response.

Figure 5.41 Osteochondritis dissecans of the right medial femoral condyle.

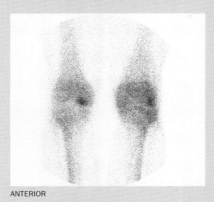
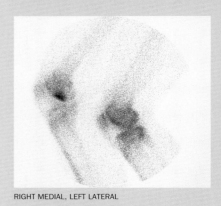

ANTERIOR

RIGHT MEDIAL, LEFT LATERAL

Figure 5.42 Osteochondritis dissecans of the medial femoral condyle. Fluid surrounds the separated fragment.

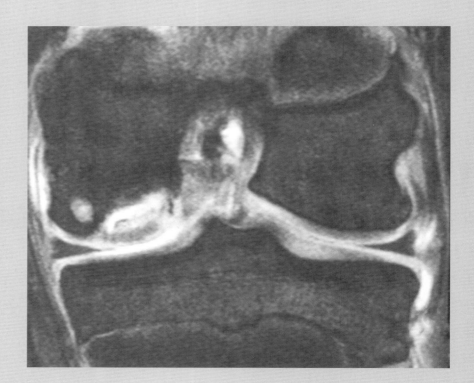

Menisci

The bone scan has been advocated by some authors as useful in detecting meniscal tears, the SPECT views purporting to show the sites of tears in the menisci (or the injury at the cartilage/bone interface). The technique has not gained wide clinical acceptance and the MRI scan is the preferred imaging method in this condition.

Other conditions (Figs 5.43–5.46)

Many other conditions can cause pain around the knee. Some examples with positive bone scan findings are included. Non-sporting causes should always be kept in mind.

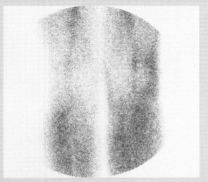

ANTERIOR BLOOD POOL

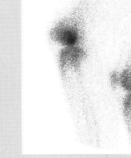

ANTERIOR

Figure 5.43 Soft tissue contusion lateral to the left knee. While there is extensive soft tissue uptake on both the blood pool and delayed images, there is no significant increase in bony uptake. The scan was performed to exclude fracture.

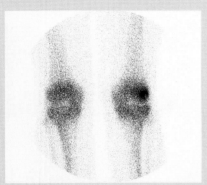

ANTERIOR

LEFT LATERAL, RIGHT MEDIAL

Figure 5.44 Osteoid osteoma in the left lateral femoral condyle. Note that the focus of uptake is not at the articular surface but deeper in the condyle. Patients presenting as sporting injuries may have non-sporting pathology.

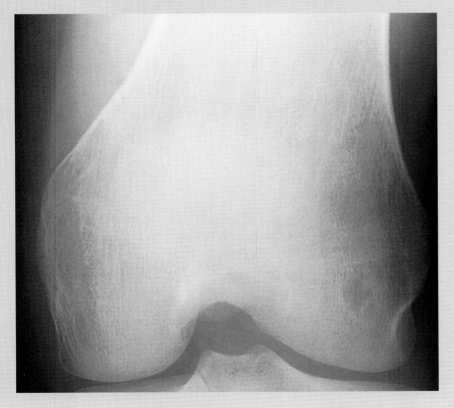

Figure 5.45 Marrow expansion. In many haematological disorders, there may be peripheral expansion or infiltration of bone marrow, commonly seen around the knees. This may be a cause of obscure knee pain. Note the prominent diffuse increase in uptake in the femoral and tibial condyles.

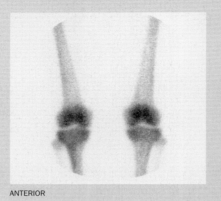

ANTERIOR

Figure 5.46 Right knee reconstruction in the post-operative phase. Note the increased uptake in the right tibia at the site of tunnelling.

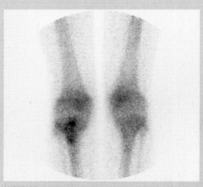

ANTERIOR

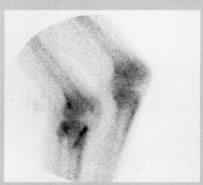

RIGHT LATERAL, LEFT MEDIAL

Bibliography

Collier BD, Johnson RP, Carrera GF, Isitman AT, Veluvolu P, Knobel J, Hellman RS, Barthelemy, CR, Chronic knee pain assessed by SPECT: comparison with other imaging modalities, *Radiology* 157: 1985, pp 795–802

Cook, GJR, Ryan, PJ, Clarke, SEM, Fogelman, I, SPECT bone scintigraphy of anterior cruciate ligament injury, *J Nucl Med*, 37: 1996, pp 1353–6

Etchebehere, EC, Etchebehere, M, Gamba, R, Belangero, W, Camargo, E, Orthopedic pathology of the lower extremities: scintigraphic evaluation of the thigh, knee and leg, *Seminars in Nuc Med* 28: 1998, pp 41–61

Fertakos, RJ, Swayne, LC, Colston, WC, Three-phase bone imaging in bone marrow edema of the knee, *Clin Nucl Med* 20: 1995, pp 587–90

Marks, PA, Goldenberg, JA, Vezina, WC, Chamberlain, MJ, Vellet, D, Fowler, PJ, Subchondral bone infractions in acute ligamentous knee injuries demonstrated on bone scintigraphy and magnetic resonance imaging, *J Nucl Med* 33: 1992, pp 516–20

Mosar, P, Gregg, J, Jacobstein, J, Radionuclide imaging in internal derangements of the knee, *Am J Sports Med* 15: 1987, pp 132–7

Murray, IP, Dixon, J, Kohan, L, SPECT for acute knee pain, *Clin Nucl Med* 15: 1990, pp 828–40

Rockett, JF, Magill, HL, Moinuddin, M, Buchignani, JS, Scintigraphic manifestation of iliotibial band injury in an endurance athlete, *Clin Nucl Med*, 16: 1991, pp 836–8

6 The pelvis, hip and thigh

The pelvis is the powerhouse of the body's musculo-skeletal system, with big muscle groups affording stability and at the same time having the ability to provide explosive power to the sprint athlete. The hips are sturdy, and stable joints and extraordinary loads are transmitted across their weightbearing areas during sporting activities. In spite of this robust role, sporting injuries in the pelvis and hip are relatively uncommon. Nevertheless, problems do occur and when the hip and groin are involved, the injury can be of career-threatening importance and is often difficult to diagnose. Imaging is usually required, either to confirm a clinical suspicion or, in the more complex cases, to help determine the underlying process.

The bone scan is a valuable diagnostic tool, particularly in the more obscure cases. As in all nuclear medicine examination, the anatomical region above and below the symptomatic site is imaged. This means that, in this particular region, the examination extends from the spine to the knee. This is important because it allows those unexpected and distant causes of referred pain to be discovered.

Tips on technique

The views usually acquired are:

· Anterior and posterior views of the pelvis;
· Oblique views, both anterior and posterior, can be invaluable in accurately locating pathology or excluding artefacts;
· Caudal or subpubic view—used to separate radioactive urine in the bladder from uptake in the symphysis pubis;
· Lumbar views—when imaging the spine, the best planar images are obtained with the patient seated and the spine flexed so that the camera is close to the spine and not distanced by a lumbar lordosis. SPECT spinal views may be helpful;
· Femoral views;
· Anterior knee views—if an abnormality is noted, laterals should be obtained;
· Lateral pelvic views;
· Anterior view with caudal tilt (camera pressing on the abdomen) may help separate bladder activity from the symphysis pubis (Fig. 6.1).

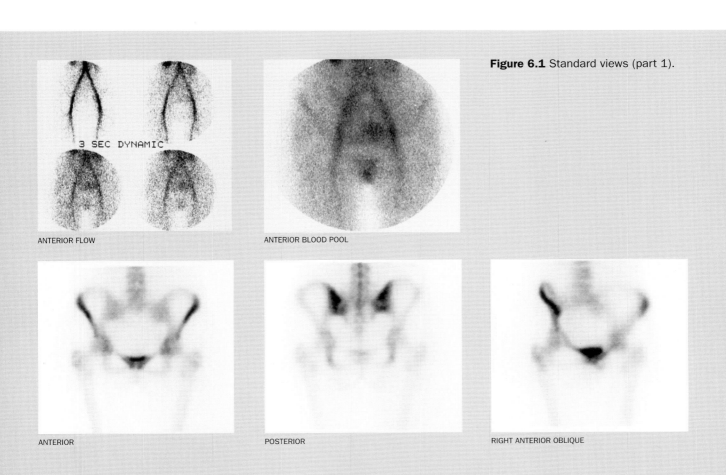

Figure 6.1 Standard views (part 1).

ANTERIOR FLOW

ANTERIOR BLOOD POOL

ANTERIOR

POSTERIOR

RIGHT ANTERIOR OBLIQUE

Figure 6.1 Standard views (part 2).

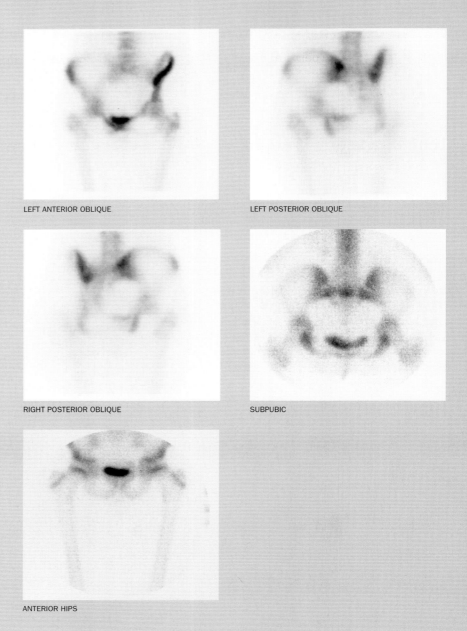

LEFT ANTERIOR OBLIQUE

LEFT POSTERIOR OBLIQUE

RIGHT POSTERIOR OBLIQUE

SUBPUBIC

ANTERIOR HIPS

Fractures (Figs 6.2–6.12)

Acute fractures of the pelvis and hip are rare in sport. Trauma associated with high-speed activities like skiing, equestrian events and contact sports will occasionally produce fractures in this region. Also, when mishaps occur in high-risk activities like parachuting and rock-climbing, major trauma can obviously be expected. Coccygeal fractures may occur with lesser trauma. Bone scans are particularly valuable when subtle or occult fractures are undetected by plain radiography. Occult fractures are most often seen following a fall and may involve the pelvic ring (usually the pubic rami and the sacroiliac joint), the sacrococcygeal region, the greater trochanter and femoral neck. These are more commonly seen in the older age group and are often insufficiency fractures.

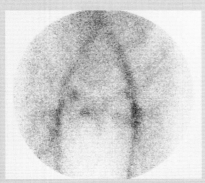

ANTERIOR BLOOD POOL

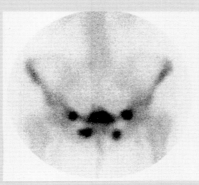

ANTERIOR

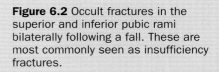

Figure 6.2 Occult fractures in the superior and inferior pubic rami bilaterally following a fall. These are most commonly seen as insufficiency fractures.

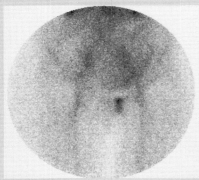

ANTERIOR BLOOD POOL

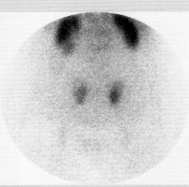

POSTERIOR BLOOD POOL

Figure 6.3 Pelvic ring fractures. The early and delayed views show increased vascularity and uptake of isotope in both sacroiliac joints and in the left side of the symphysis pubis. The early views are very important because pubic fractures may be obscured by radioactive urine in the bladder in the delayed images. Note how the subpubic view helps separate the pubic bones from the bladder.

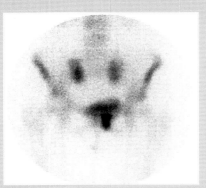

ANTERIOR

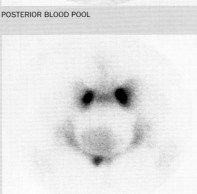

SUBPUBIC

Figure 6.4 'H' fracture in the sacrum and fracture in the right side of the symphysis pubis. The subpubic view shows that the activity on the left side of the symphysis is due to urine in the bladder. The greatest activity in the sacral insufficiency fracture is along the sacroiliac joints, with lesser uptake across the midsacrum.

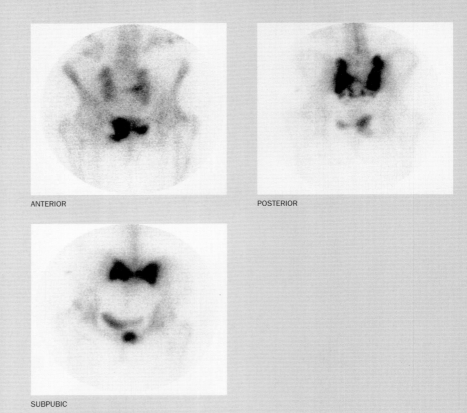

ANTERIOR

POSTERIOR

SUBPUBIC

Figure 6.5 Oblique fracture of the right ilium and pelvic ring fractures involving the sacroiliac joints, sacrum, left superior and inferior pubic rami and the left side of the symphysis pubis. The iliac fracture is less commonly seen than the pelvic ring fractures.

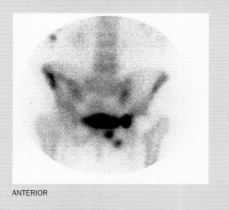

ANTERIOR

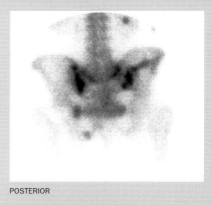

POSTERIOR

Figure 6.6 Fracture of a spinous process in the upper sacrum. Planar and SPECT views demonstrate a focal area of increased uptake in a spinous process in the upper sacrum due to fracture.

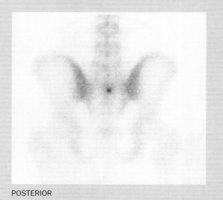

POSTERIOR

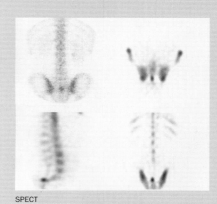

SPECT

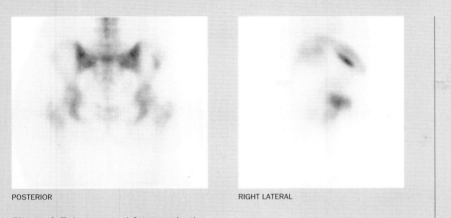

POSTERIOR

RIGHT LATERAL

Figure 6.7 An unusual fracture in the right iliac bone laterally below the crest, due to a fall on the right side.

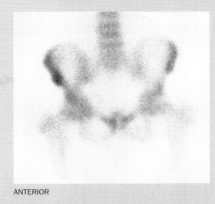

ANTERIOR

Figure 6.8 Avulsion fracture of the right anterior superior iliac spine at the origin of the sartorius muscle.

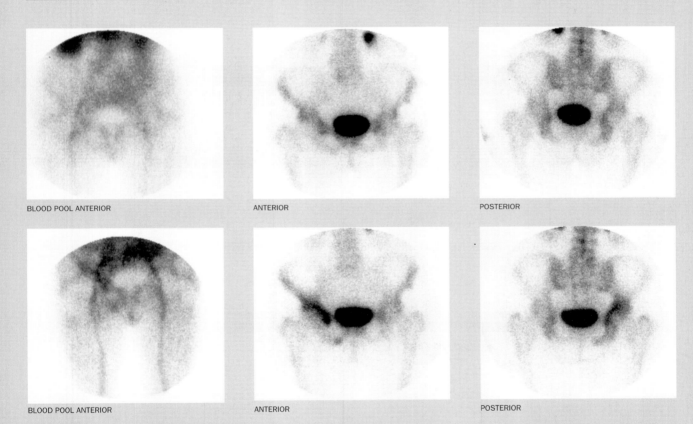

BLOOD POOL ANTERIOR

ANTERIOR

POSTERIOR

BLOOD POOL ANTERIOR

ANTERIOR

POSTERIOR

Figure 6.9 Evolution of changes due to fracture in the right acetabulum on two studies performed 7 days apart. The first study (top row) shows minimal increase in uptake in the right acetabulum. The second study (bottom row) shows the more typical appearance of acetabular fracture, with increase on both the blood pool and delayed images. It is important to note that the scan changes due to fracture may not be evident in the first few days after trauma, particularly in the elderly and osteoporotic. Focal hyperaemia early after trauma may be the only sign of fracture.

Figure 6.10 Occult fracture in the neck of the left femur. This fracture was due to a fall rather than repetitive stress.

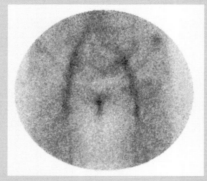

BLOOD POOL ANTERIOR

ANTERIOR

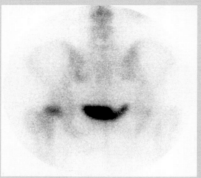

POSTERIOR

Figure 6.11 Occult fracture in the neck of the left femur due to a fall. Note that there is avascularity of the left femoral head.

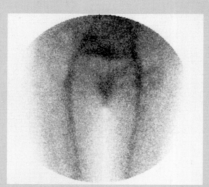

BLOOD POOL ANTERIOR

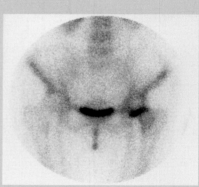

ANTERIOR

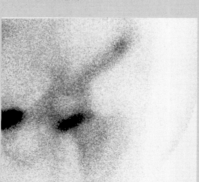

ANTERIOR ZOOM

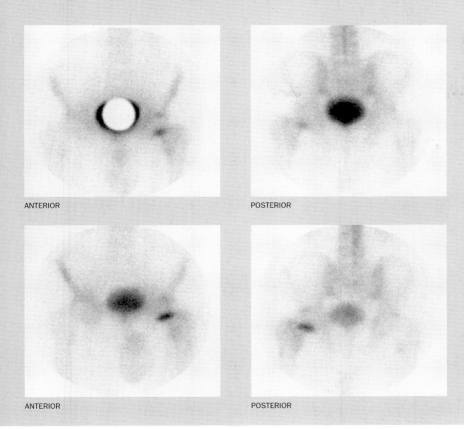

Figure 6.12 Left femoral neck fracture demonstrating evolution of the fracture over time. The first study (top row) 2 days after a fall shows mild uptake at the inferior edge of the femoral neck. The second study (bottom row) was performed 9 days later and demonstrates more typical changes of fracture.

ANTERIOR

POSTERIOR

ANTERIOR

POSTERIOR

Apophyseal avulsion injuries are common around the pelvis and the hip joint in immature athletes. The vast majority of these are the result of overuse, rather than caused purely by a single muscle contraction. There is invariably a history of pain and disability localised to the area for a few days or weeks prior to the avulsion occurring. If the athlete were investigated at this early stage, chronic stress would produce increased uptake at the apophyseal growth plate.

Avulsion injuries also occur in the mature athlete, most commonly involving the ischial tuberosity (Figs 6.13–6.15).

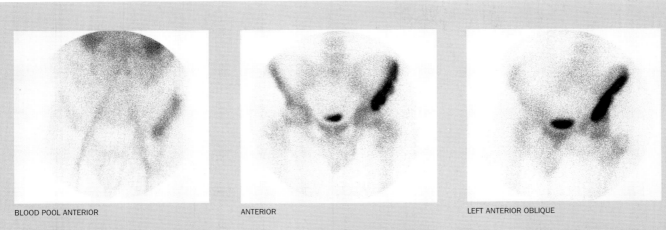

BLOOD POOL ANTERIOR

ANTERIOR

LEFT ANTERIOR OBLIQUE

Figure 6.13 Left iliac apophyseal fracture. There is intense increase in blood flow and uptake in the left iliac crest anteriorly due to an acute avulsion fracture of the apophysis incurred during weightlifting.

Figure 6.14 Irregularity of the margins of the ischial apophysis indicates apophysitis. There has also been slight avulsion of the apophysis. The left hip shows dysplastic features.

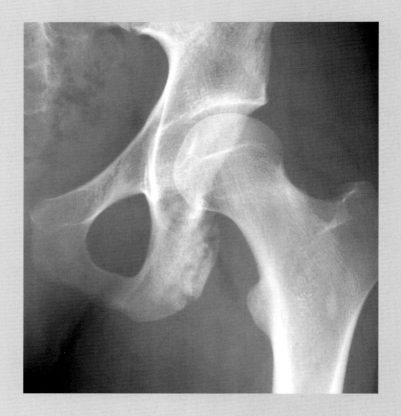

Figure 6.15 Hamstring avulsion in an Olympic hurdler.

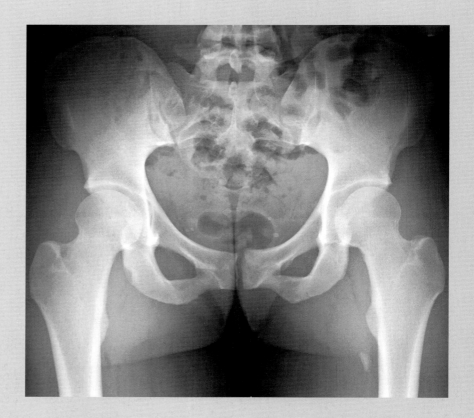

Bone stress and stress fractures are less common in the pelvis and hip than elsewhere in the lower limbs (Figs 6.16–6.20).

The most important site is the neck of femur. The stress changes usually occur at the base of the femoral neck on the inferior or compressive side. Fractures may also involve the superior or traction side but these are characteristically seen in the older age group, are usually insufficiency fractures and are rare in athletes. Classical dance, long-distance running and hiking have an increased incidence of femoral neck stress fractures. Pinning of these fractures is sometimes necessary to prevent progression to a complete fracture and to help avoid the complications of non-union and avascular necrosis. Bone scans are highly sensitive in detecting this condition and the authors consider that some of the literature on this subject is misleading.

Shin et al., in assessing MRI as a method for imaging and diagnosing femoral neck stress fractures, reported a series of 19 military recruits with 22 'stress fractures'. They all had hip pain, normal plain films and positive bone scans. The changes seen on MRI showed that five of the 22 were false positives and the uptake in these cases was due to a synovial pit, an iliopsoas tear, bilateral iliopsoas tendinitis, an obturator internus tendinitis and, in one case, possible early AVN. The conclusion drawn was that MRI should be the investigation of choice for the diagnosis of femoral neck stress fractures, being 100% accurate, whereas bone scan has an accuracy of 68% with a false positive rate of 32%. The authors feel that the accuracy of bone scan for the diagnosis of this condition approaches 100% and, had oblique views of the pelvis been taken, then the uptake anterior and posterior to the hip would have been projected away from the femoral neck and the false positives avoided. The increased uptake associated with the synovial pit may have been the only true false positive, but this would also have been difficult to interpret on MRI, where the differentiation from an intracapsular osteoid osteoma would have been difficult. A few false negatives for both modalities have been reported.

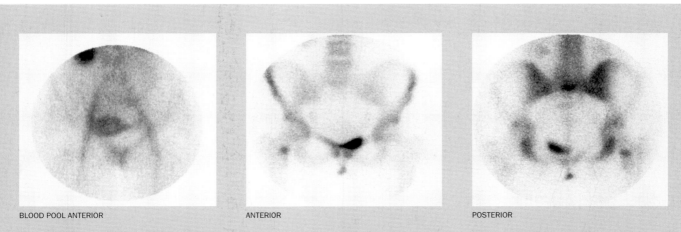

BLOOD POOL ANTERIOR   ANTERIOR   POSTERIOR

Figure 6.16 Stress fracture in the inferior edge of the right femoral neck. This is the commonest site of stress fracture in the femoral neck.

Figure 6.17 A fracture line appearing in an area of bone stress. Linear low density in the right femoral neck indicates that trabecular fractures have coalesced to produce a linear fracture, which at this stage is incomplete.

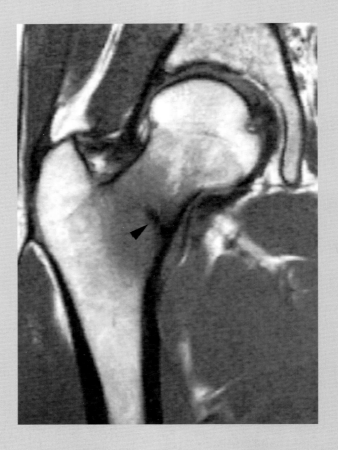

Figure 6.18 There is a stress fracture on the compressive side of the femoral neck. Cystic change, a sign of poor prognosis, is demonstrated (arrow).

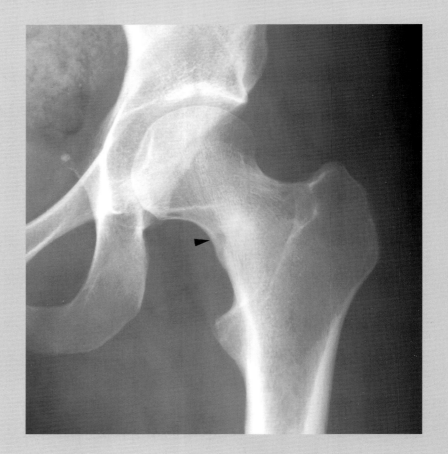

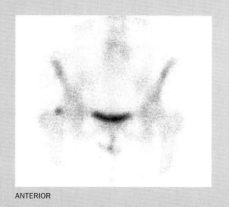
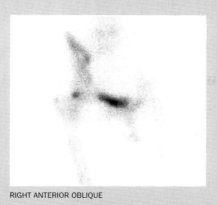

ANTERIOR

RIGHT ANTERIOR OBLIQUE

Figure 6.19 Stress fracture in the superior surface of the right femoral neck. Stress fractures at this site are more commonly seen in the older age group.

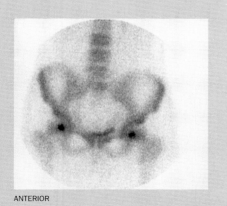
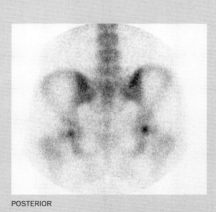

ANTERIOR

POSTERIOR

Figure 6.20 Bilateral femoral head stress fractures. These are less common than femoral neck stress fractures in the authors' experience, and may occur medially or laterally in the femoral head.

Stress fractures of the pubic rami occur most commonly in female middle- and long-distance runners. Bone mineral density should always be assessed, as these fractures are often insufficiency fractures. Noak et al. used the characteristic clinical presentation of this condition to make the clinical diagnosis and bone scans to confirm the findings. Bone scans enable the diagnosis to be made prior to plain film changes appearing (Figs 6.21–6.24).

Figure 6.21 Fracture of the right inferior pubic ramus. The focal increase in uptake of isotope in the right inferior pubic ramus represents a stress fracture at this site.

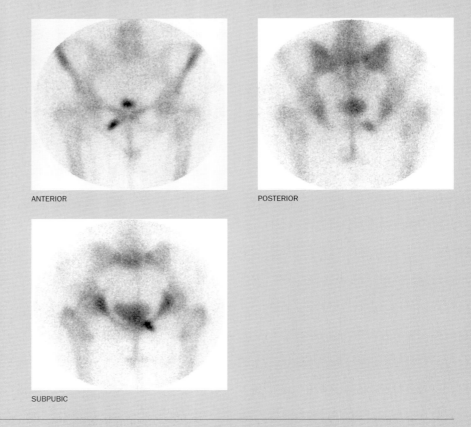

ANTERIOR

POSTERIOR

SUBPUBIC

Figure 6.22 Stress fractures of pubic rami occur more commonly in female athletes and are often associated with low bone density.

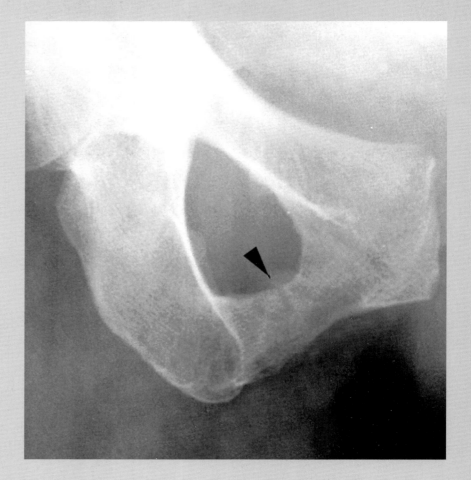

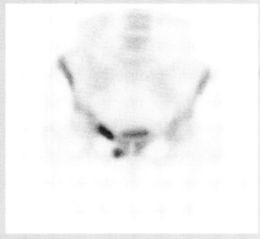

ANTERIOR

Figure 6.23 Stress fractures involving the right superior and the inferior pubic rami have developed along a linear plane of stress. The changes are shown on the anterior bone scan image and on plain film. (Images courtesy of Dr R Highet.)

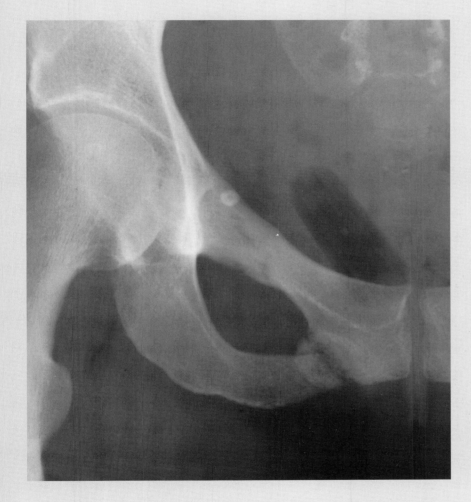

Figure 6.24 Left ischiopubic synchondrosis. This is a common normal finding in young patients and should not be confused with fracture.

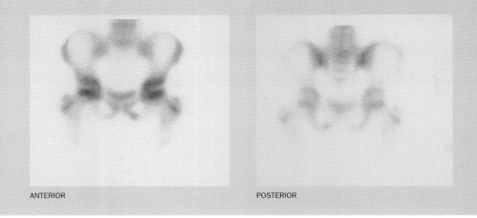

ANTERIOR POSTERIOR

Stress fractures also involve the sacrum. This condition is seen almost exclusively in athletes who compete or train over long distances. A decreased bone density should be considered in the female athlete (Fig. 6.25).

Figure 6.25 Stress fracture of the sacrum in a 14-year-old athlete shown by bone scan and CT scan.

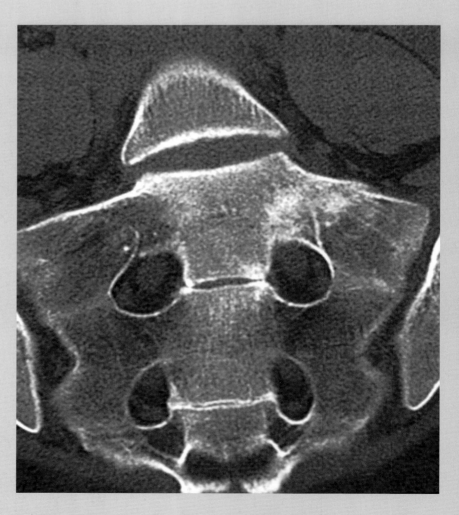

POSTERIOR

The femoral shaft is occasionally the site of bone stress, seen mainly in the elite athlete. Bone stress in the subtrochanteric region and midshaft usually presents with what appears to be muscle ache. The changes may be demonstrated in the characteristic pattern of cortical involvement. On MRI some cases show high signal confined to the medulla. Supracondylar stress reaction is commonly seen in long-distance runners and is more likely to progress to a stress fracture than the more proximal sites of bone stress (Figs 6.26 and 6.27).

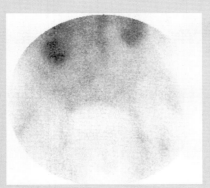

BLOOD POOL ANTERIOR

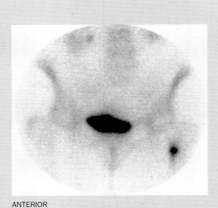

ANTERIOR

Figure 6.26 Stress fracture in the proximal left femur just below the lesser trochanter.

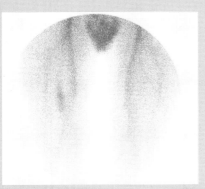

BLOOD POOL ANTERIOR

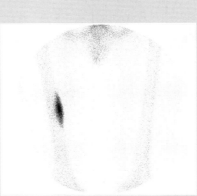

ANTERIOR

Figure 6.27 Stress fracture in the midshaft of the right femur medially.

A further condition occurring as the result of stress is slipping of the capital femoral epiphysis. This is a chronic process disrupting the growth plate of the femoral head that, if untreated, may result in inferomedial slipping of the epiphysis. Before displacement occurs the process can be detected on a bone scan and a positive scan may precede plain radiological changes. These early changes are detected as asymmetry of uptake in the growth plate on both the early blood pool and delayed images. This is obviously the optimal time to diagnose the condition and early investigation is encouraged. In performing the scan, rigid attention to technique is required. There must be symmetrical positioning of the feet (best with heels apart and toes together) so that varied rotation of the hips won't be misinterpreted as asymmetry. Using 'frogleg' views will usually produce optimal images of the growth plate, and pinhole images should also be performed to improve resolution (Figs 6.28–6.30).

Figure 6.28 Right slipped capital femoral epiphysis. The blood pool images demonstrate increased vascularity in the right femoral neck growth plate compared to the left. This is often the most sensitive indicator of this condition. The delayed image shows increased uptake in the right growth plate.

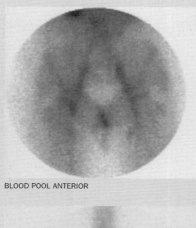
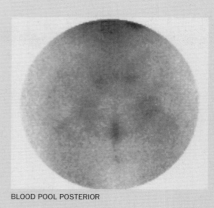

BLOOD POOL ANTERIOR

BLOOD POOL POSTERIOR

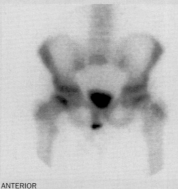

ANTERIOR

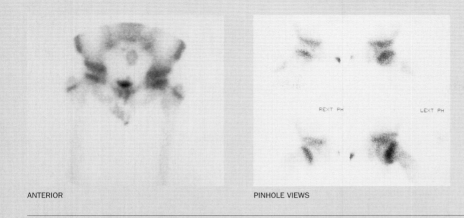

ANTERIOR   PINHOLE VIEWS

Figure 6.29 Left slipped capital femoral epiphysis. The planar image shows a subtle increase in uptake throughout the left hip and in the growth plate. The pinhole views demonstrate increased uptake across the left capital femoral growth plate, best demonstrated in external rotation (bottom row). Activity in the joint itself may be due to secondary synovitis or, if severe, chondrolysis.

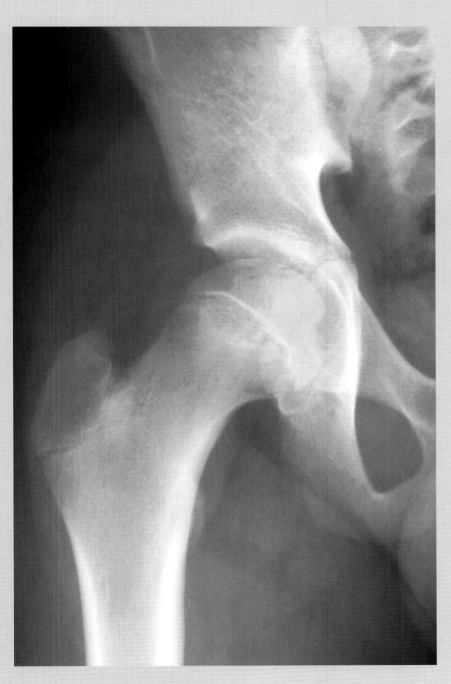

Figure 6.30 Early slipping of the epiphysis of the right femoral head.

Arthritis (Figs 6.31–6.35)

Degenerative joint changes involving the spine, pelvis and hips are often seen as an incidental finding. In the sporting population these degenerative changes may be the result of previous sports-related injury and in the ageing athlete are so common that they are almost 'normal' findings. The clinical significance of these changes is sometimes difficult to determine. The more intense the uptake, the more likely it is to be clinically relevant. The imaging results must always be considered with the clinical picture. It is important to remember that hip and groin pain may be due to degenerative changes in the lumbar spine.

Inflammatory arthritis may present in the sporting population and when a diffuse synovitis is seen in the hip or sacroiliac joint, this diagnosis should be considered.

Figure 6.31 Arthritis in the right hip. Increased uptake of isotope is seen in the articular surface of the right hip, extending throughout the capsule due to arthritis. A line of activity across the femoral neck anteriorly may be seen when capsulitis is present and should not be misinterpreted as a fracture. Uptake over the left greater trochanter is due to trochanteric bursitis. Note the oblique artefacts due to fat folds.

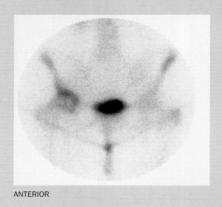

ANTERIOR

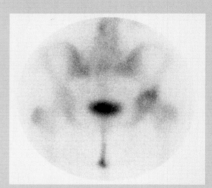

POSTERIOR

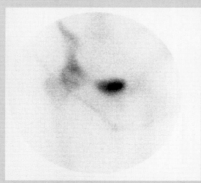

RIGHT ANTERIOR OBLIQUE

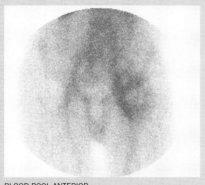

BLOOD POOL ANTERIOR

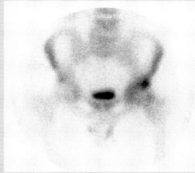

ANTERIOR

Figure 6.32 Severe arthritis in the left hip. Early and delayed views show increased blood flow and uptake of isotope throughout the left hip joint due to arthritis, with more focal uptake at the superior acetabular lip due to osteophyte formation.

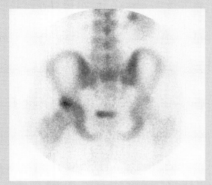

POSTERIOR

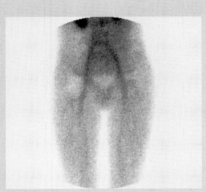

BLOOD POOL ANTERIOR

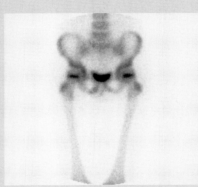

ANTERIOR

Figure 6.33 Transient synovitis in the right hip. The reduction in blood pool activity in the right hip is due to a large effusion. The delayed images are almost normal, with the pinhole images showing only a subtle increase in uptake in the right acetabulum.

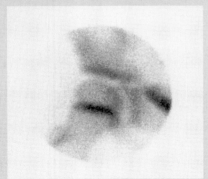

RIGHT PINHOLE

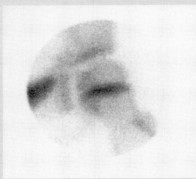

LEFT PINHOLE

161

Figure 6.34 Bilateral sacroiliitis. There is focal increase in uptake in both sacroiliac joints inferiorly at the synovial surface.

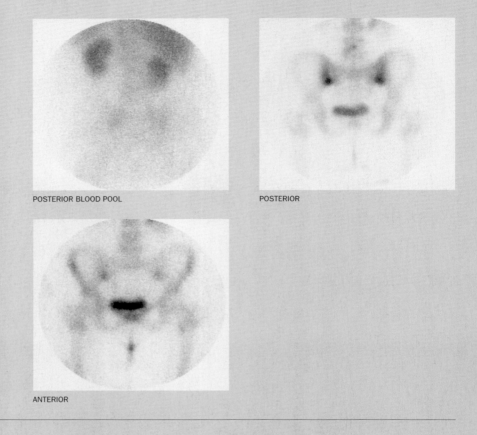

POSTERIOR BLOOD POOL

POSTERIOR

ANTERIOR

Figure 6.35 Bilateral sacroiliitis. There is increased blood flow and uptake of isotope throughout the sacroiliac joints, more marked on the left side. This appearance is more commonly seen in inflammatory arthritis.

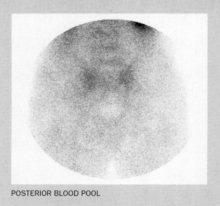

POSTERIOR BLOOD POOL

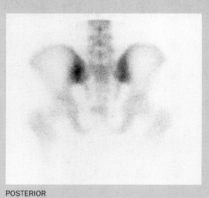

POSTERIOR

Enthesopathy, tendinosis and bursitis

These processes, usually produced by repetitive stress, may occur independently or coexist and are most commonly detected at the greater trochanter, lesser trochanter, ischial tuberosity, pubic region and at the anterior inferior iliac spine. A bone scan is very sensitive to the bony disruption and repair of an enthesopathy and is the most sensitive technique for detection of abnormality at the bone/tendon interface.

The soft tissue changes of tendinitis and bursitis cannot be consistently and dependably demonstrated by bone scan. These processes may occasionally be seen on delayed images but are mostly seen during the blood pool phase of a bone scan. Consequently, MRI and ultrasound are the preferred methods of imaging of these soft tissue changes (Fig. 6.36).

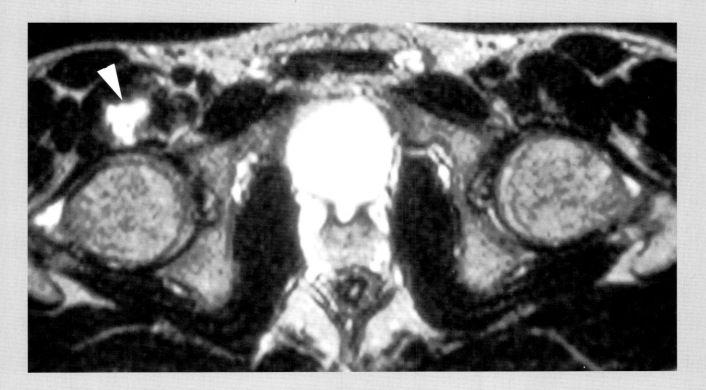

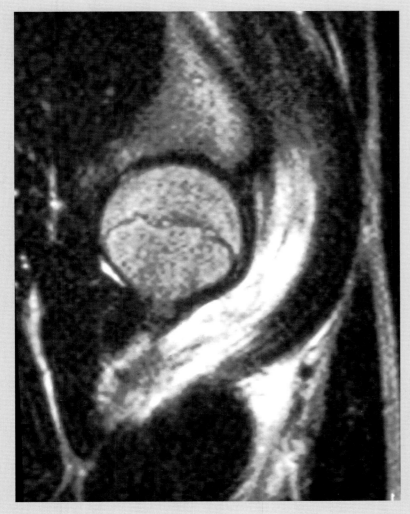

Figure 6.36 Left iliopsoas tendinopathy demonstrated by MRI in both the axial (arrow) and sagittal planes.

Greater trochanter (Figs 6.37–6.44)

Enthesopathy at the greater trochanter may be associated with the insertion of the gluteus medius, gluteal minimus, vastus lateralis and the piriformis, although often the exact origin of uptake is difficult to define. Enthesopathy, tendinitis and trochanteric bursitis often coexist when associated with chronic aetiological factors such as a leg-length discrepancy, poor running biomechanics or lumbar degenerative disease. Occasionally, calcification can be seen on plain films, indicating associated tendinitis. The authors have noted that symptoms produced by these processes at the greater trochanter are often misinterpreted as pain originating from the hip joint or spine.

Figure 6.37 Mild left trochanteric bursitis/gluteal insertion enthesopathy. In this case the abnormality is the typical line of increased uptake vertically over the greater trochanter. The blood pool image was normal.

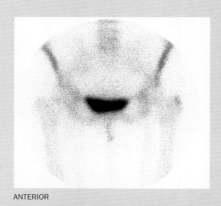

ANTERIOR

Figure 6.38 Bilateral trochanteric bursitis/gluteal enthesopathy. The blood pool and delayed views show increased vascularity and uptake in the characteristic site.

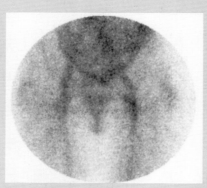

BLOOD POOL ANTERIOR

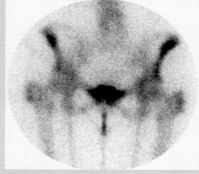

ANTERIOR

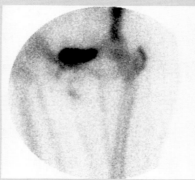

LEFT ANTERIOR OBLIQUE

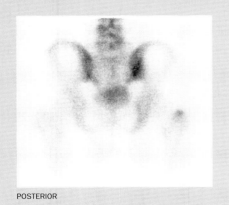

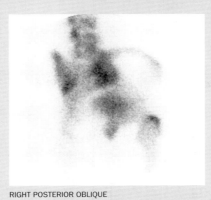

POSTERIOR

RIGHT POSTERIOR OBLIQUE

Figure 6.39 Right piriformis enthesopathy.

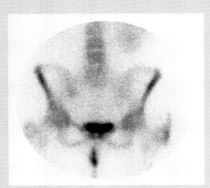

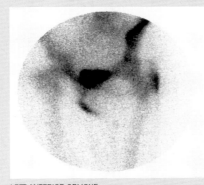

ANTERIOR

LEFT ANTERIOR OBLIQUE

Figure 6.40 Left gluteal tendinitis and trochanteric bursitis. Note how the increase in uptake extends from the muscle insertion site into the soft tissue adjacent to the greater trochanter, along the line of gluteal muscles.

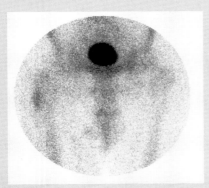

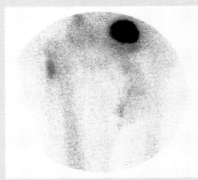

ANTERIOR

RIGHT ANTERIOR OBLIQUE

Figure 6.41 Vastus lateralis tendinitis and enthesopathy.

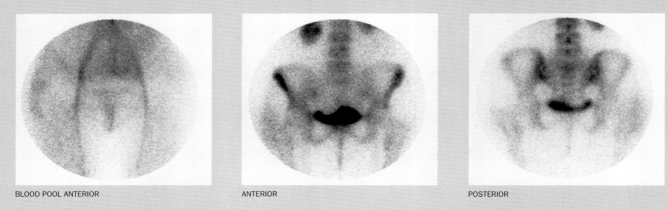

BLOOD POOL ANTERIOR   ANTERIOR   POSTERIOR

Figure 6.42 Soft tissue contusion over the right greater trochanter following a fall. The early and delayed views show soft tissue uptake with no bony abnormality.

Figure 6.43 Gluteus muscle injury in the right buttock. There is soft tissue uptake extending from the right iliac crest to the greater trochanter along the line of the muscle. No bony pathology was evident.

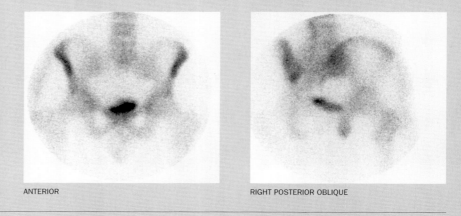

ANTERIOR   RIGHT POSTERIOR OBLIQUE

Figure 6.44 Left iliac crest enthesopathy and gluteal muscle injury. There is soft tissue uptake in the left buttock due to muscle injury, with a small focal area of increased uptake in the iliac crest at the site of muscle origin.

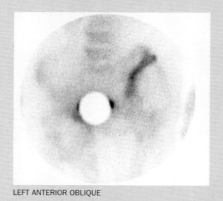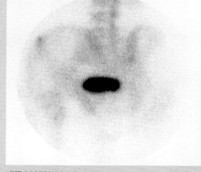

LEFT ANTERIOR OBLIQUE   LEFT POSTERIOR OBLIQUE

Lesser trochanter (Figs 6.45–6.47)

Enthesopathy at the insertion of the iliopsoas tendon produces a focus of increased uptake at the lesser trochanter. Iliopsoas tendinosis is rarely seen on bone scan and MRI or ultrasound are the preferred methods for the demonstration of iliopsoas tendinosis.

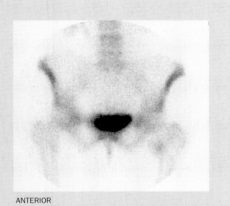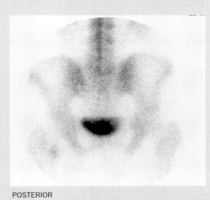

ANTERIOR   POSTERIOR

Figure 6.45 Enthesopathy at the iliopsoas muscle insertion in the lesser trochanter of the left femur.

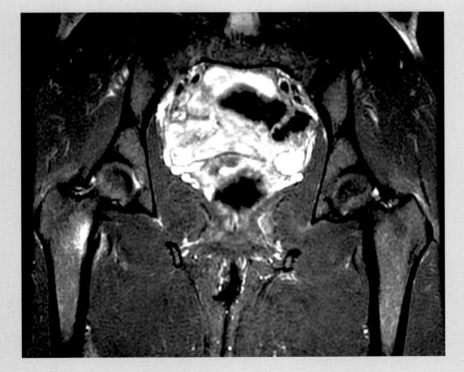

Figure 6.46 Right iliopsoas enthesopathy.

Figure 6.47 Enthesopathy in the proximal left femur. There is periostitis in the left femur just below the lesser trochanter due to enthesopathy at the insertion of the iliopsoas or the pectineus.

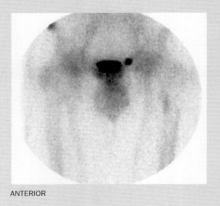

ANTERIOR

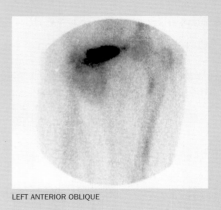

LEFT ANTERIOR OBLIQUE

Groin (Figs 6.48–6.54)

Bone scans are a valuable tool in the complex minefield of groin pain. When the groin pain is due to a distant process, such as the lumbar spine or hip, a bone scan is ideal, as a large anatomical area is covered by the examination. Local causes including enthesopathy at the insertion of the adductor tendons, osteitis pubis, or enthesopathy at the insertion of the conjoint tendon/inguinal ligament are well demonstrated on bone scan. There is often more than one cause present due to a progressive instability that appears to characterise the condition and it is important that, having found a possible cause of groin pain, other coexisting causes, such as a hernia, are excluded.

Thus if the pathology is at the insertion site, the bone scan is very sensitive. Optimal imaging is essential and requires complete emptying of the bladder just prior to imaging. Encouraging extra fluid intake between the early and delayed views is also useful so that residual urine in the bladder is dilute. It is also important to have the collimator in close proximity to the pelvis by tilting the camera head. If the bladder still overlies the pubis, then either a subpubic image or anterior view with caudal tilt may provide separation.

Figure 6.48 Right adductor insertion enthesopathy. There is mild increase in uptake of isotope in the right inferior pubic ramus at the site of adductor muscle insertion.

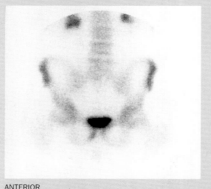

ANTERIOR

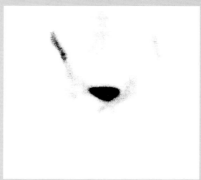

RIGHT ANTERIOR OBLIQUE

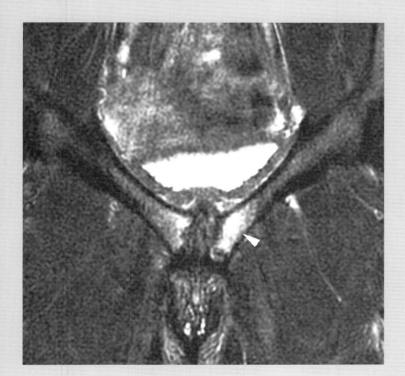

Figure 6.49 Left adductor enthesopathy associated with osteitis pubis (arrow).

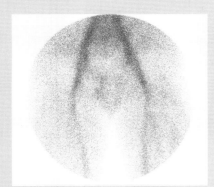

BLOOD POOL ANTERIOR

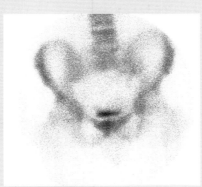

ANTERIOR

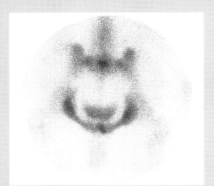

SUBPUBIC

Figure 6.50 Right osteitis pubis. There is focal increase in uptake of isotope in the right side of the symphysis pubis extending to the pubic tubercle. The early view shows a mild increase in blood flow on the right side. The aetiology of this appearance is most likely adductor enthesopathy.

Figure 6.51 Right pubic tubercle enthesopathy. There is a mild focal increase in vascularity and uptake in the right pubic tubercle at the insertion of the conjoint tendon/inguinal ligament.

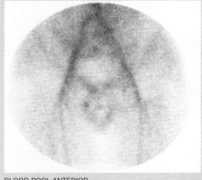

BLOOD POOL ANTERIOR

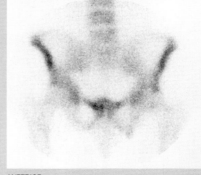

ANTERIOR

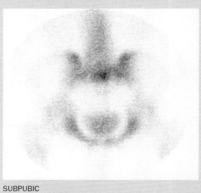

SUBPUBIC

Figure 6.52 Pubic symphysitis. There is increased uptake of isotope extending symmetrically across the symphysis pubis. Note that the vascularity on the blood pool images is not in the symphysis but is pudendal.

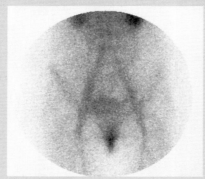

BLOOD POOL ANTERIOR

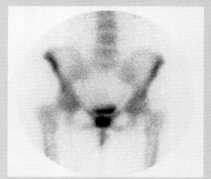

ANTERIOR

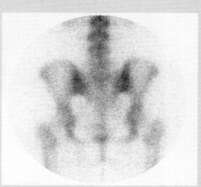

POSTERIOR

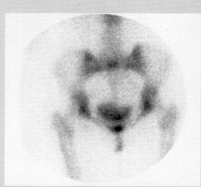

SUBPUBIC

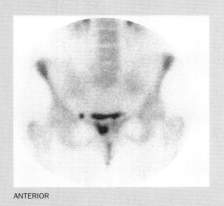

ANTERIOR

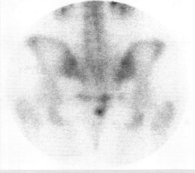

POSTERIOR

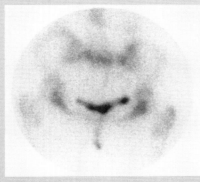

SUBPUBIC

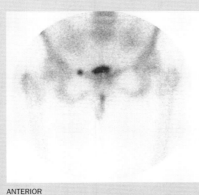

ANTERIOR

Figure 6.53 Bladder artefact simulating pathology in the symphysis pubis. The initial anterior and posterior images (top row) suggest the presence of abnormality in the right side of the symphysis pubis with a further focus in the right superior pubic ramus. The subpubic view shows no abnormal uptake in the symphysis or pubic rami and demonstrates that radioactive urine in the bladder accounts for the activity at both sites. A repeat post-void anterior view (bottom row) demonstrates the normal pubic symphysis. The patient's hip pain was due to the mild right greater trochanter enthesopathy. This case demonstrates the care needed to exclude urinary artefacts simulating pubic pathology.

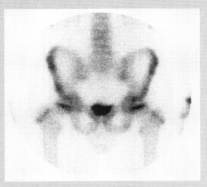

ANTERIOR

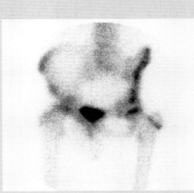

LEFT ANTERIOR OBLIQUE

Figure 6.54 Enthesopathy at the origin of the right rectus femoris muscle at the anterior inferior iliac spine. The changes are subtle and the oblique views help confirm the asymmetry.

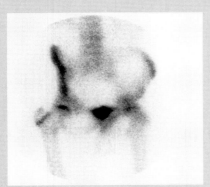

RIGHT ANTERIOR OBLIQUE

Ischial tuberosity (Figs 6.55–6.58)

Pain and tenderness at the ischial tuberosity may be due to a muscle or tendon tear, tendinosis of one or more of the hamstring tendons, with or without an associated enthesopathy. Bursae are also found at the ischial tuberosity and bursitis is thought to be a cause of pain in this region. The blood pool images may show local hypervascularity, especially if there is a large degree of soft tissue change. When enthesopathy is a major component of the process, delayed images will show significant uptake. Posterior oblique views of the pelvis may be helpful.

Figure 6.55 Bilateral hamstring enthesopathy/ischial bursitis. Increased uptake is noted in both ischial tuberosities. The oblique views are useful in this condition.

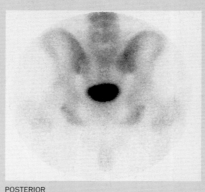

POSTERIOR

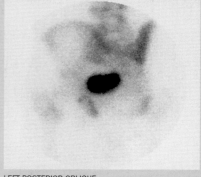

LEFT POSTERIOR OBLIQUE

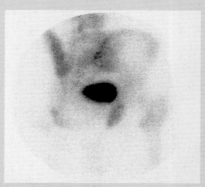

RIGHT POSTERIOR OBLIQUE

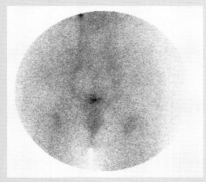

POSTERIOR BLOOD POOL

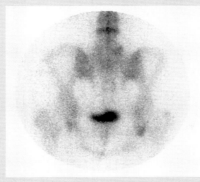

POSTERIOR

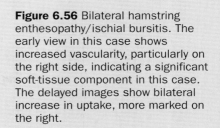

Figure 6.56 Bilateral hamstring enthesopathy/ischial bursitis. The early view in this case shows increased vascularity, particularly on the right side, indicating a significant soft-tissue component in this case. The delayed images show bilateral increase in uptake, more marked on the right.

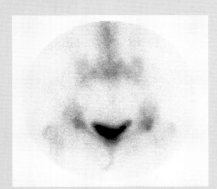

SUBPUBIC

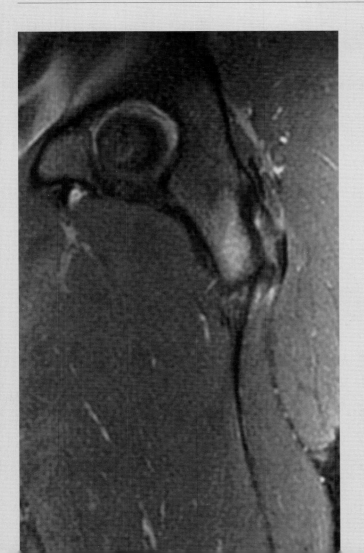

Figure 6.57 Enthesopathy at the left ischial tuberosity due to recurrent hamstring traction.

Figure 6.58 Severe left hamstring insertion enthesopathy.

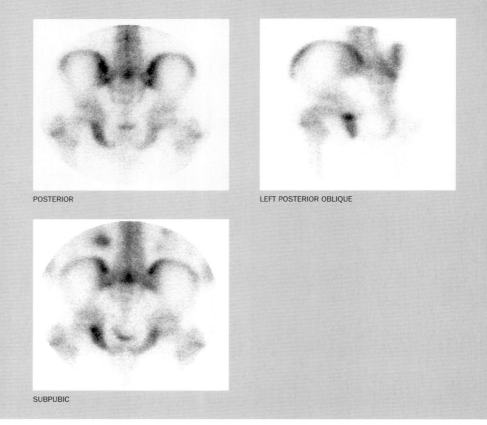

POSTERIOR

LEFT POSTERIOR OBLIQUE

SUBPUBIC

Thigh splints (Figs 6.59–6.62)

This is the term given to a diffuse form of bone stress in the femur. Stress may occur as the result of loading due to excessive muscular action resulting in remodelling. This may be the consequence of poor technique and is often associated with jumping sports. It has also been described in short-legged female army recruits following strenuous marching. Thigh pain can be severe. We have also seen it as an incidental finding. The bone scan has a characteristic appearance of linear uptake usually on the lateral border of the femur and seen only on the delayed images. The flow study and early view are normal in this condition. If the condition is of long standing, cortical hypertrophy may be apparent on plain films.

Figure 6.59 Periosteal reaction in the mid left femoral shaft laterally due to enthesopathy at the origin of the vastus muscles. This abnormality is often termed 'thigh splints'. Usually, there is no abnormal uptake in the blood pool image, but a linear band of uptake is seen at the muscle/bone interface on the delayed images.

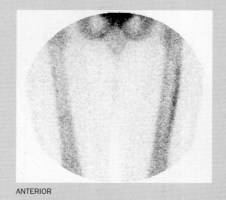

ANTERIOR

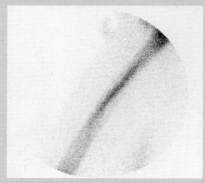

LEFT LATERAL

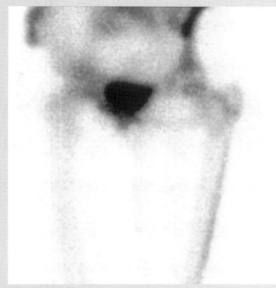

LEFT ANTERIOR OBLIQUE

Figure 6.60 Left 'thigh splint'. The bone scan image shows cortical or periosteal uptake along the left femoral shaft laterally. Plain films show lateral cortical hypertrophy in the left femur. This is the take-off leg of a highjumper.

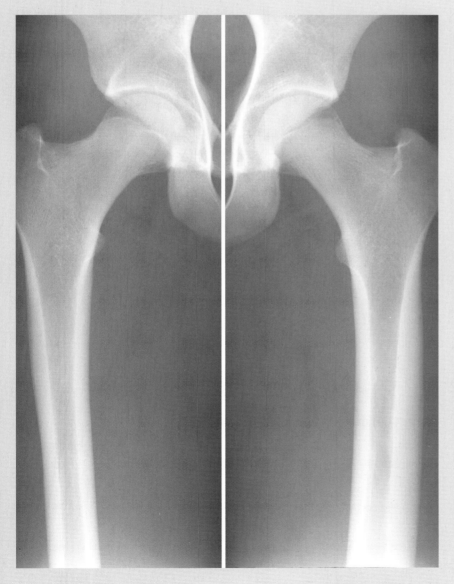

Figure 6.61 Bilateral periosteal reaction (thigh splints) in the femurs. The left is worse than the right.

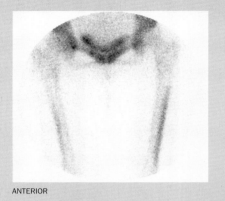

ANTERIOR

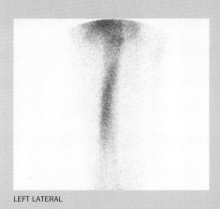

LEFT LATERAL

Figure 6.62 Enthesopathy in the proximal left femur posterolaterally. This may be at the insertion of the gluteus maximus or at the origin of the vastus lateralis.

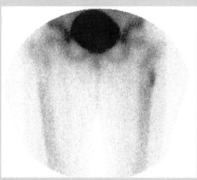

ANTERIOR

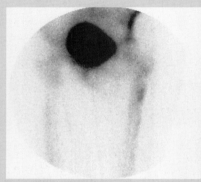

LEFT ANTERIOR OBLIQUE

Muscle injury (Figs 6.63–6.68)

Muscle injury is best demonstrated by ultrasound or MRI. On bone scans, acute muscle injury may show hyperaemia on the blood pool images. Uptake may also be seen in the muscle on the delayed views due to altered calcium metabolism in the damaged muscle. Uptake in the later stages may be due to the formation of heterotopic calcification.

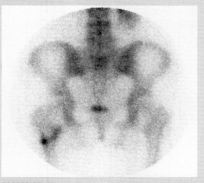

POSTERIOR

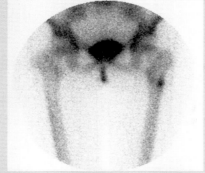

ANTERIOR

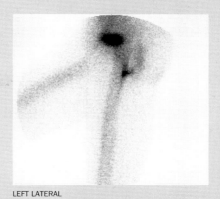

LEFT LATERAL

Figure 6.63 Muscle tear with calcification in soft tissue extending from a femoral fracture. The lateral view is essential to demonstrate the soft tissue component.

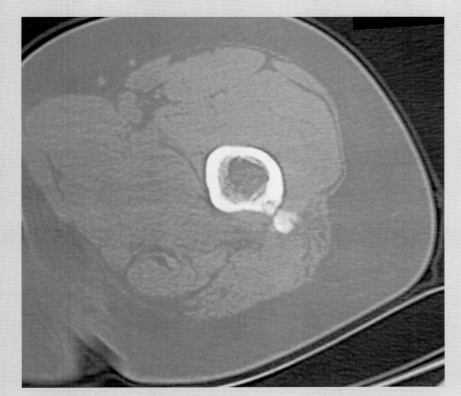

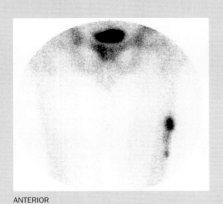

ANTERIOR

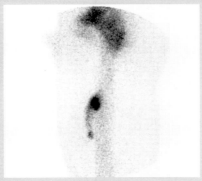

LEFT LATERAL

Figure 6.64 Left vastus intermedius muscle tear with unusual soft tissue uptake.

Figure 6.65 Left hamstring tear well demonstrated by ultrasound. MRI shows a tear in the medial hamstring.

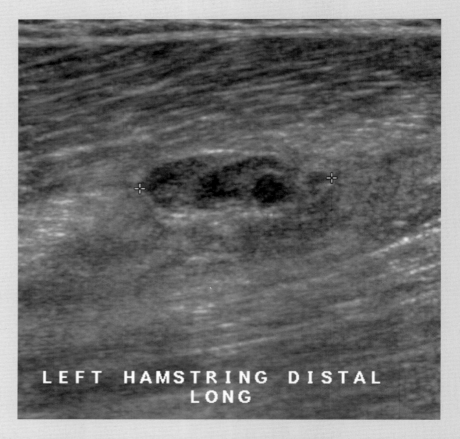

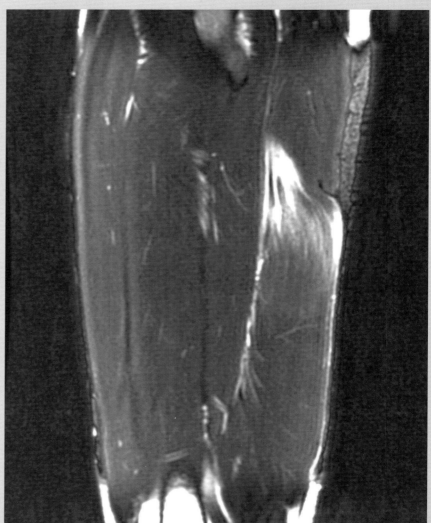

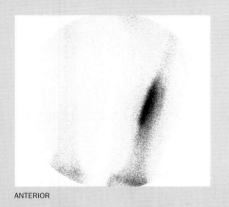
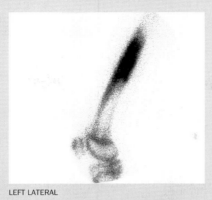

ANTERIOR   LEFT LATERAL

Figure 6.66 Severe acute periosteal tear in a sprinter. There is extensive uptake along the insertion of the left vastus intermedius muscle. Subsequent imaging showed only very mild calcification anterior to the femur, but no fracture was seen.

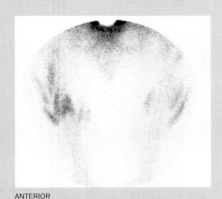

ANTERIOR

Figure 6.67 Multiple intramuscular injections in the anterior thighs. Any cause of muscle trauma may induce focal uptake at the site.

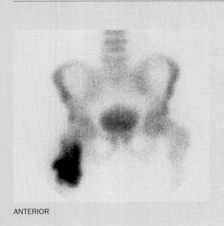
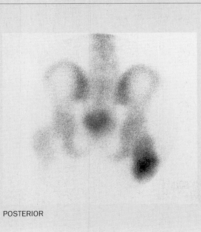

ANTERIOR   POSTERIOR

Figure 6.68 Heterotopic bone formation anterior to the proximal right femur. This occurred following recent spinal injury with paraplegia.

Avascular necrosis of the femoral head (Figs 6.69–6.73)

Most causes of avascular necrosis of the femoral head are beyond the scope of this book. The condition occurs spontaneously in adults or presents as a complication of corticosteroid therapy and the use of anabolic steroids.

Avascular necrosis of the femoral head may also occur as a consequence of a femoral neck fracture or resulting from nitrogen embolism from scuba diving.

In children, the condition of Perthes' disease is spontaneously occurring avascular change in the femoral head epiphysis. Avascular necrosis may also be a complication of slipped femoral head epiphysis.

Early in the avascular process, absent or reduced uptake may be observed in the femoral head. As the disease progresses and revascularisation occurs, increase in uptake is then seen in the femoral head.

Figure 6.69 Avascular necrosis in the left femoral head. There is a small focus of increased uptake superolaterally in the head of the left femur due to avascular necrosis.

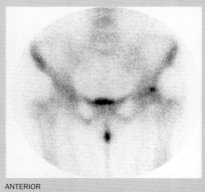
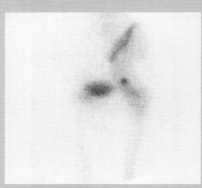

ANTERIOR

LEFT ANTERIOR OBLIQUE

Figure 6.70 Avascular necrosis in the right femoral head. There is increased uptake in the subarticular region of the head of the right femur, indicating avascular necrosis in the revascularising phase. Note that the uptake does not extend into the acetabulum.

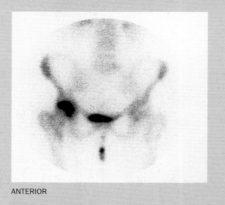
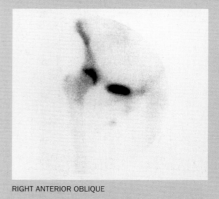

ANTERIOR

RIGHT ANTERIOR OBLIQUE

Figure 6.71 Segmental avascular necrosis of the left femoral head superiorly. In the early phase there is a 'cold' segment with increased uptake at the margins.

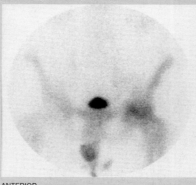

ANTERIOR

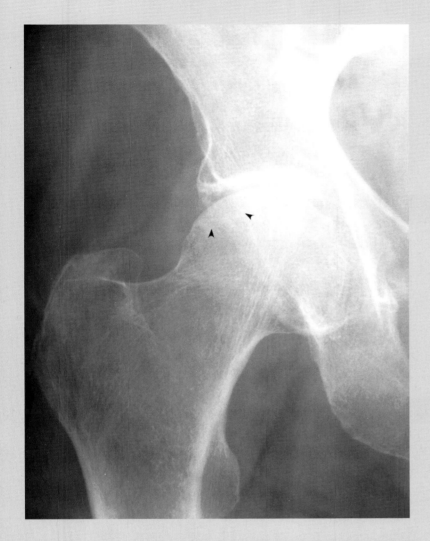

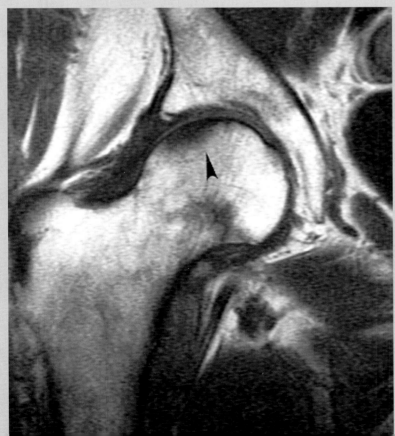

Figure 6.72 Avascular necrosis of the femoral head shown on plain film. There is localised subchondral demineralisation (arrows). MRI clearly demonstrates the area of avascular change (arrow).

Figure 6.73 Perthes' disease of the left hip. Pinhole views are usually necessary to obtain optimal views of the hips in this condition.

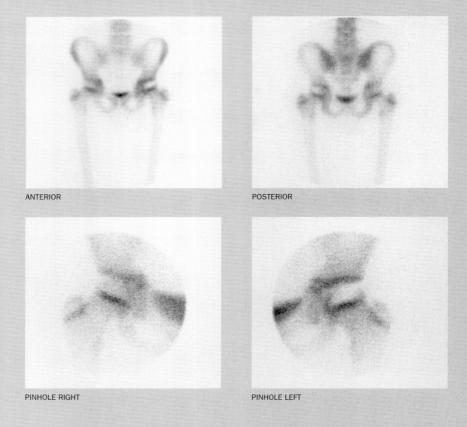

ANTERIOR

POSTERIOR

PINHOLE RIGHT

PINHOLE LEFT

Bibliography

Allwright, SJ, Cooper, RA, Nash, P, Trochanteric bursitis: bone scan appearance, *Clin Nucl Med* 13: 1988, pp 561–4

Amako, T, Kawashima, M, Torisu, T, Hayashi, K, Bone & joint lesions in decompression sickness, *Semin Arthritis Rheum* 4: 1974, pp 151–90

Briggs, RG, Kolbjornses, PH, Southhall, RC, Osteitis pubis, Tc-99m MDP, and professional hockey players, *Clin Nucl Med* 17: 1992, pp 861–3

Casey, D, Mirra, J, Staple, TW, Parasymphyseal insufficiency fractures of the os pubis, *AJR* 142: 1984, pp 581–6

Collier, BD, Carrera, GF, Johnson, RP, Isitman, AT, Hellman, RS, Knobel, J, Finger, WA, Gonyo, JE, Malloy, PJ, Detection of femoral head avascular necrosis in adults by SPECT, *J Nucl Med* 26: 1985, pp 979–87

Cooper, KL, Beabout, JW, Swee, RG, Insufficiency fractures of the sacrum, *Radiology* 156: 1985, pp 15–20

Devas, MB, Stress fractures of the femoral neck, *J Bone Joint Surg* [Br] 47: 1965, pp 728–38

Erne, P, Burkhardt, A, Femoral neck fatigue fracture, *Arch Orthop Traumat Surg* 97: 1980, pp 213–20

El-Khoury, GY, Wehbe, M, Bonfiglio, M, Chow, KC, Stress fractures of the femoral neck: a scintigraphic sign for early diagnosis, *Skeletal Radiol* 6: 1981, pp 271–3

Gelfand, MJ, Streiffe, JL, Graham, EJ, Bone scintigraphy in slipped capital femoral epiphysis, *Clin Nucl Med* 8: 1983, pp 613–15

Holder, LE, Machin, J, Asdourian, PL, Links, JM, Sexton, CC, Planar and high resolution SPECT bone imaging in the diagnosis of facet syndrome, *J Nucl Med* 36: 1995, pp 37–44

Holder, LH, Schwarz, C, Wernicke, PG, Michael, RH, Radionuclide bone imaging in the early detection of fractures of the proximal femur (hip): multifactorial diagnosis, *Radiology* 174: 1990, pp 509–15

Keene, JS, Lash, EG, Negative bone scan in femoral neck stress fracture. A case report, *Am J Sports Med* 20, 1992, pp 2324–6

Kim, SM, Park, CH, Gartland, JJ, Stress fracture of the pubic ramus in a swimmer, *Clin Nucl Med* 12: 1987, pp 118–19

Khoury, MB, Kirks, DR, Martinez, S, Apple, J, Bilateral avulsion fractures of the anterior superior iliac spines in sprinters, *Skeletal Radiol* 13: 1985, pp 65–7

Koch, RA, Jackson, DW, Pubic symphysitis in runners, A report of two cases, *Am J Sports Med* 9: 1981, pp 349–58

Kujala, UM, Orava, S, Karpakka, J, Leppavuori, J, Mattila, K, Ischial tuberosity apophysitis and avulsion among athletes, *Int J Sports Med* 18: 1997, pp 149–55

Metzmaker, JN, Pappas, AM, Avulsion fractures of the pelvis, *Am J Sports Med* 13: 1985, pp 349–58

Meurman, KOA, Stress fracture of the pubic arch in military recruits, *Br J Radiol* 53: 1980, pp 521–4

Noak, TD, Smith, JA, Lindenberg, G, Wills, CE, Pelvic stress fractures in long distance runners, *Am J Sports Med* 13: 1985, pp 120–3

O'Connor, MK, Brown, ML, Hung, JL, Hayostek, RJ, The art of bone scintigraphy—technical aspects, *J Nucl Med* 32: 1991, pp 2332–41

Pres, T, Detection of osteoporotic sacral fractures with radionuclides, *Radiology* 146: 1983, pp 783–5

Shin, AY, Morin, WD, Gorman, JD, Jones, SB, Lapinsky, AS, The superiority of magnetic resonance imaging in differentiating hip pain in endurance athletes, *Am J Sports Med* 24: 1996, pp 168–76

Tyler, JL, Derbekyan, V, Lisbona, R, Early diagnosis of myositis ossificans with Tc-99M diphosphonate imaging, *Clin Nucl Med* 9: 1984, pp 256–8

Volpin, G, Milgrom, C, Goldsher, D, Stein, H, Stress fractures of the sacrum following strenuous activity, *Clin Ortho* 243: 1999, pp 184–8

Wiley, JJ, Traumatic osteitis pubis—the gracilis syndrome, *Am J Sports Med* 11: 1983, pp 360–3

7 The spine

The spine is constantly stressed in all sporting pursuits. There is commonly a combination of axial loading, twisting movements with lateral or anterior flexion and extension. Each position of the spine is counteracted by muscle and ligamentous forces. This means that wear and tear on the spine will be seen as both soft tissue and bony injury. Superimpose on this chronic repetitive trauma and the violent effect of contact sports, and the high frequency of spinal problems in athletes is easy to understand.

Not only is back pain very common in athletes but is a common complaint in the general community. Consequently, sporting activity may in fact not be the cause of some back pain but rather aggravate a pre-existing spinal problem.

Because of the complexity of the anatomy of the spine, there is great dependency on bone scans as a sensitive technique in the diagnosis of occult fractures, bone stress and stress fractures. Bone scans may also be helpful in the evaluation of degenerative processes in the apophyseal joints.

Tips on technique

Both planar and SPECT imaging are usually required in the examination of the spine. Ideally, planar imaging is best performed with the patient seated and positioned with their back flexed and resting directly against the camera. Good oblique views can also be obtained in this position (Fig. 7.1). Imaging through a low attenuation bed, with the patient supine and without flexion, will result in inferior images. Occasionally this may be the only option in an incapacitated patient.

SPECT imaging can be performed with a 360-degree or 180-degree acquisition and the patient may be prone or supine. Each method has its advocates. 360-degree SPECT with the patient supine is probably the most popular method. Reconstruction is usually obtained in the transaxial, sagittal and coronal planes. Oblique reconstruction in the plane of the spine around the area of interest has been advocated by some and may improve localisation.

The SPECT scan has been shown to be more sensitive for the detection of bone stress and stress fractures than is planar imaging. When the planar scan is normal, the SPECT scan should still be performed because of its higher sensitivity. If the planar scan is abnormal, the SPECT study will still be used because of its ability to accurately localise the area of uptake. Lumbar SPECT has been well documented to be beneficial, although its use in the cervical and thoracic region is still being assessed.

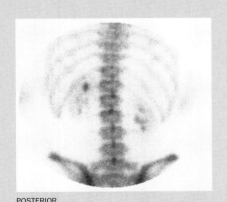
POSTERIOR

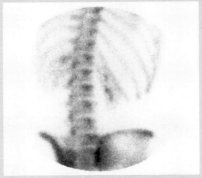
RIGHT POSTERIOR OBLIQUE

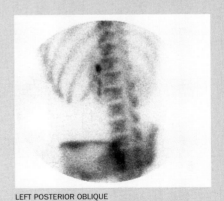
LEFT POSTERIOR OBLIQUE

Figure 7.1 Normal views of the lumbar spine. These views were obtained with the patient seated with the lumbar spine flexed and resting against the surface of the gamma camera. Note the good separation of the vertebral bodies.

Choice of imaging method

In the investigation of back pain, plain radiography is the first line imaging investigation. Plain films can provide considerable information and are particularly useful in excluding the unexpected finding such as a bone tumour or an aortic aneurysm as the cause of the back pain.

A bone scan is the next investigation in athletes with a suspected occult fracture and is particularly useful when there is a clinical presentation suggestive of bone stress or a stress fracture. The presence of other occult fractures, such as fractures of spinous or transverse processes, will also become apparent on a bone scan. Bone scans have a very different mechanism of action from plain radiography and CT, and can be helpful in evaluating the significance of pathology seen on these studies. For example, bone scan may help assess whether a pars defect or facet joint degeneration is clinically significant and the cause of symptoms.

CT is the next investigation of choice if bone detail is important to demonstrate or if soft tissue or bony encroachment on the spinal canal is thought likely. Disc protrusions and disc encroachment on exit foramina are well shown by CT and, with the availability of the multislice image acquisition, CT's role in the investigation of the spine will further expand.

MRI has a specialist role in the investigation of spinal problems. This modality is used to assess spinal injury where injury to the cord may have occurred and is especially valuable in the assessment of functional spinal stenosis in the cervical spine. Cervical and thoracic discs are much more easily seen on MRI images and the presence of abnormal signal in lumbar discs is easily detected.

Where possible the plain films, CT and MRI studies should be viewed simultaneously with the bone scan. Not only will valuable diagnostic information be available, enabling a more informative report to be made, but essential information such as the presence of transitional vertebrae or previous surgery may be brought to light. Not all referring doctors include such significant information on a consultation form and not all patients remember or consider these important facts relevant.

Fractures (Figs 7.2–7.11)

Occult fractures in the spine occur due to either direct trauma or transmitted force and may involve the vertebral bodies, transverse processes or posterior elements.

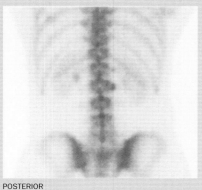

POSTERIOR

SPECT TRANSAXIAL

SPECT CORONAL

SPECT SAGITTAL

Figure 7.2 Fracture of the right transverse process of the L2 vertebra. Planar and SPECT images show increased uptake in the transverse process. A lesser degree of uptake is also evident on the planar image in the right transverse process of L1. This injury was caused by a knee to the back during a rugby match.

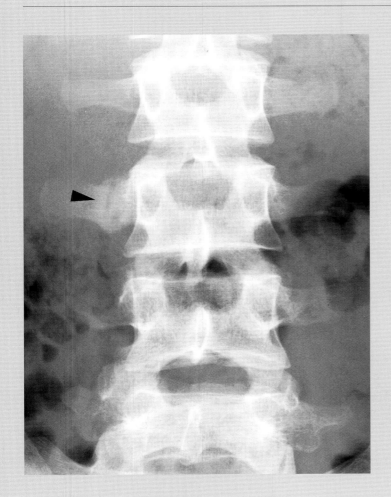

Figure 7.3 Stress fracture of a transverse process in a professional dancer (arrow).

Figure 7.4 Fracture of the spinous process of T2. The blood pool, delayed planar and SPECT images show a focal increase in uptake due to recent traumatic fracture.

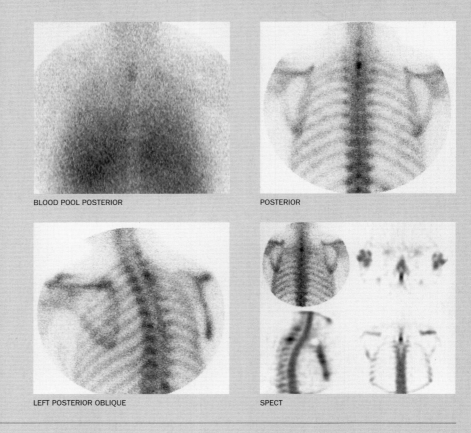

BLOOD POOL POSTERIOR

POSTERIOR

LEFT POSTERIOR OBLIQUE

SPECT

Figure 7.5 Fracture of the spinous process of the L5 vertebra demonstrated on SPECT views.

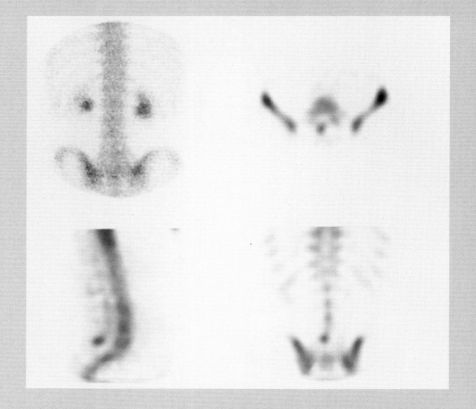

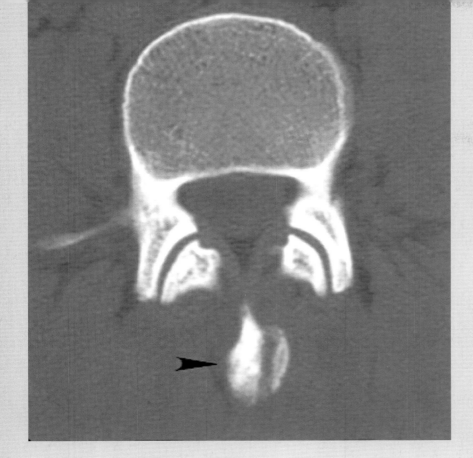

Figure 7.6 Bone stress due to a change in activity. A ballet dancer in 'Swan Lake' was required to spend long periods with a flexed lumbar spine. Traction by the interosseous ligament on the spinous process eventually produced symptomatic bone stress. The sagittal SPECT image shows stress reaction in the spinous process. The CT image shows new bone formation along the spinous process.

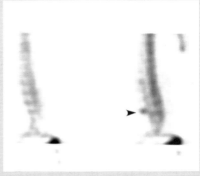

SPECT SAGITTAL

Figure 7.7 Fracture of the C4 vertebral body. While the fracture is demonstrated on the planar views in this case, SPECT views are more sensitive in the detection of lower grade fractures and also help show the extent of the fracture.

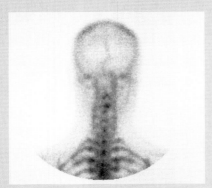

POSTERIOR

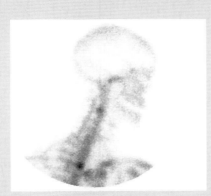

RIGHT ANTERIOR OBLIQUE

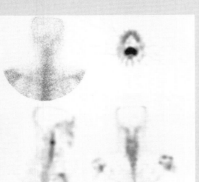

SPECT

Figure 7.8 Fracture of the superior endplate of the T12 vertebra with mild activity flaring into the vertebral body.

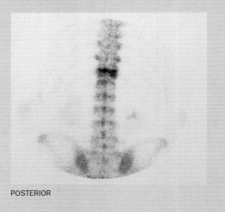

POSTERIOR

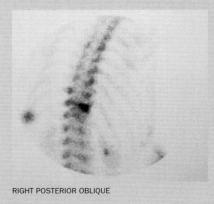

RIGHT POSTERIOR OBLIQUE

Figure 7.9 Compression fractures of the T10, T5 and T4 vertebrae. Low-grade fractures are also present in the left seventh and right ninth ribs. This appearance is most commonly seen in osteoporotic patients.

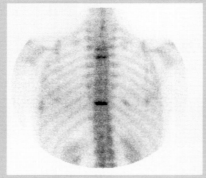

POSTERIOR

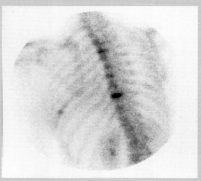

LEFT POSTERIOR OBLIQUE

Figure 7.10 Multiple occult fractures of endplates of vertebral bodies. This unusual injury occurred in a young woman who fell while skiing. Plain X-rays were initially normal, but subsequent X-rays showed evidence of fractures.

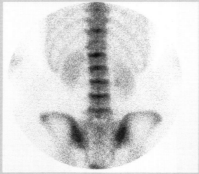

POSTERIOR

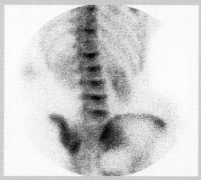

RIGHT POSTERIOR OBLIQUE

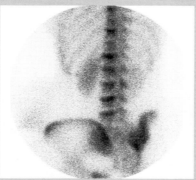

LEFT POSTERIOR OBLIQUE

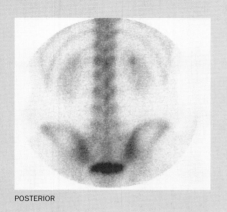

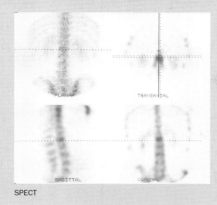

POSTERIOR   SPECT

Figure 7.11 L1 vertebral compression fracture in a late phase of healing. This fracture was imaged 8 months post-injury; however, the time frame for fracture healing on bone scans is variable.

Repetitive trauma to the spine, particularly in the lumbar region, can cause bone stress or a stress fracture at the site of maximal stress. In athletes this occurs moderately commonly at the pars interarticularis of lumbar vertebrae or less commonly in laminae, transverse or posterior spinous processes. Pars bone stress or stress fractures may be unilateral or bilateral and this appears to be determined by the mechanism of injury or the biomechanics of the sport undertaken. Unilateral changes in the pars are commonly seen in sports with a rotational component to the spinal flexion and extension, such as in fast bowling in cricket, serving in tennis and surfboard riding. Bilateral pars fractures are more commonly seen in gymnasts, in divers and in American football players where the flexion and extension are predominantly anteroposterior. Spondylolisthesis may result from bilateral pars fractures.

A pars defect demonstrated on X-ray or CT may be due to recent fracture or due to previous injury. The positive bone scan indicates active pathology (Figs 7.12–7.17).

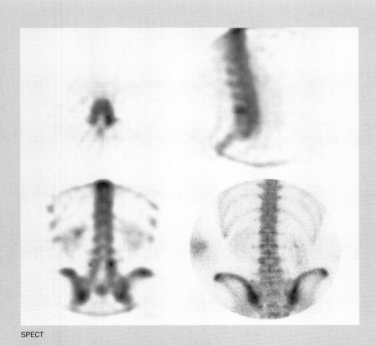

SPECT

Figure 7.12 Stress fracture of the L4 left pars interarticularis. Mild uptake is seen in the left side of L4 on the planar image. This is more obvious on the SPECT views and is localised to the pars interarticularis. Pars fractures are most commonly seen in the L4 and L5 vertebrae.

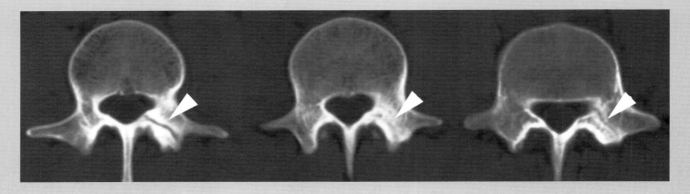

Figure 7.13 Unilateral stress fractures in a young fast bowler occurring at three different levels.

Figure 7.14 SPECT images showing fractures of the left L5 pars interarticularis and the right L4 pedicle. Note that the uptake in the L4 vertebra is more anterior and corresponds with the pedicle on the sagittal and coronal slices.

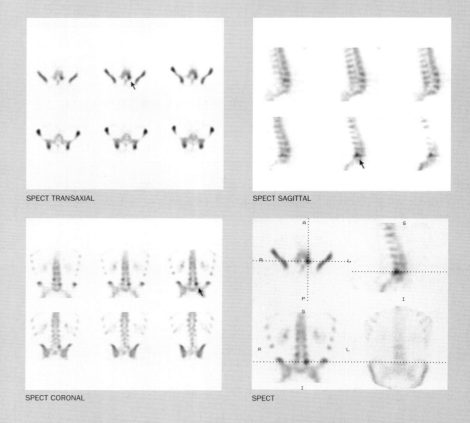

SPECT TRANSAXIAL

SPECT SAGITTAL

SPECT CORONAL

SPECT

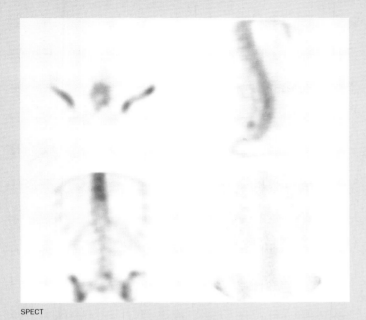

SPECT

Figure 7.15 Fracture of the left lamina of the L5 vertebra. The SPECT images show the focus of uptake is more medial on the coronal slice and more posterior on the transaxial and sagittal slices than the more common pars fracture.

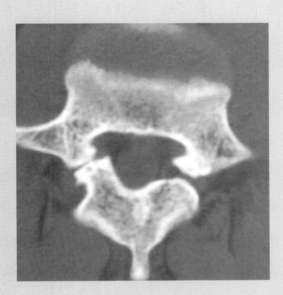

Figure 7.16 Bilateral pars interarticularis defects are present. There is established non-union and both are 'cold' on bone scan.

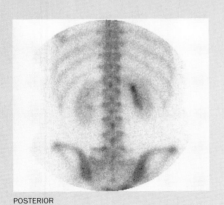

POSTERIOR   SPECT

Figure 7.17 Urine contamination. The planar image shows increased uptake on the left side of the L5 vertebra. This case demonstrates the necessity of imaging in multiple planes as the uptake was shown to be due to overlying urinary contamination in an incontinence pad on the SPECT images. Oblique or lateral images would also make this distinction.

Arthritis (Figs 7.18–7.21)

The spine is one of the common sites of degenerative change and this is often exacerbated by sports activity, particularly in older people. Anatomical imaging can show the extent of arthritis but the clinical significance will depend on bone-scan findings. Most established changes are asymptomatic. The bone scan shows sites of activity and thus provides complementary and significant information. SPECT imaging is paramount in localising the site of this activity. The demonstration of which facet joint shows increased uptake can help direct facet joint injection to the correct level.

It has been claimed that the bone scan can reliably distinguish between facet joint changes and bone stress or a stress fracture involving the pars interarticularis by the site and angulation of the increase in uptake. This has not been our experience and is not a well-accepted strength of the bone scan.

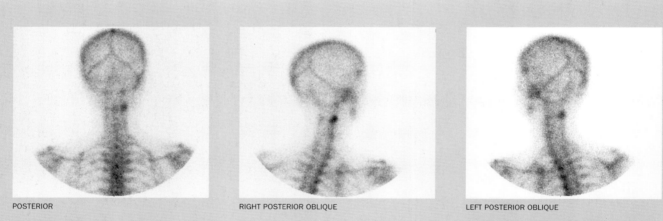

POSTERIOR   RIGHT POSTERIOR OBLIQUE   LEFT POSTERIOR OBLIQUE

Figure 7.18 Right C2/3 facet joint arthritis. This is the typical appearance of this common pathology, with focal uptake in the laterally placed facet joints in the cervical spine.

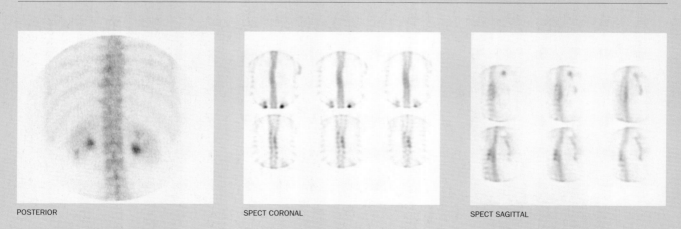

POSTERIOR   SPECT CORONAL   SPECT SAGITTAL

Figure 7.19 Facet joint arthritis in multiple lower thoracic vertebrae, more marked on the left side from T8 to T10. The SPECT images best demonstrate that the uptake is predominantly in the posterior elements due to facet joint arthritis.

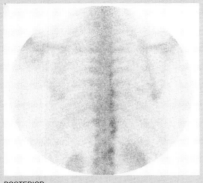

POSTERIOR

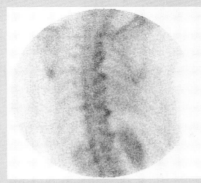

RIGHT POSTERIOR OBLIQUE

Figure 7.20 Osteophyte formation in the lower thoracic spine on the right side. The SPECT and oblique images demonstrate the uptake lies anterolateral to the vertebral bodies, indicating that this is due to osteophyte formation. It is the authors' experience that this occurs much more commonly on the right side than the left, probably related to handedness.

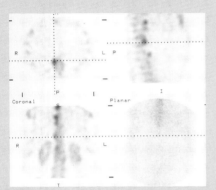

SPECT

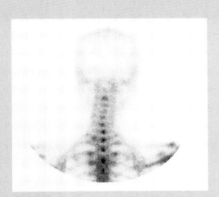

POSTERIOR

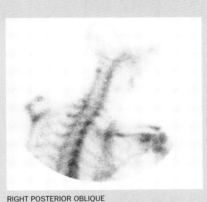

RIGHT POSTERIOR OBLIQUE

Figure 7.21 Costovertebral arthritis. Planar and SPECT images show subtle but definite focal increase in uptake of isotope in the left side of the T1 costovertebral junction. The SPECT images show the focus of uptake is more anterior than the facet joint and indicates inflammation in the demifacet for the head of the first rib.

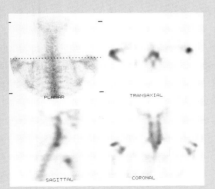

SPECT

Pseudarthrosis (Figs 7.22 and 7.23)

Occasionally a sacralised lumbar or lumbarised sacral vertebra may articulate with the sacral wing and pseudarthrosis develops. The bone scan will demonstrate uptake if secondary degenerative changes are developing and so indicate that this is likely to be the site of pain production. Post-surgical pseudarthrosis or fracture through a spinal fusion mass can similarly demonstrate increased uptake if bony activity is present.

Figure 7.22 Pseudarthrosis between a lumbarised S1 vertebra and the adjacent right sacral wing. (Images courtesy of Dr D McHarg and Dr J Burke.)

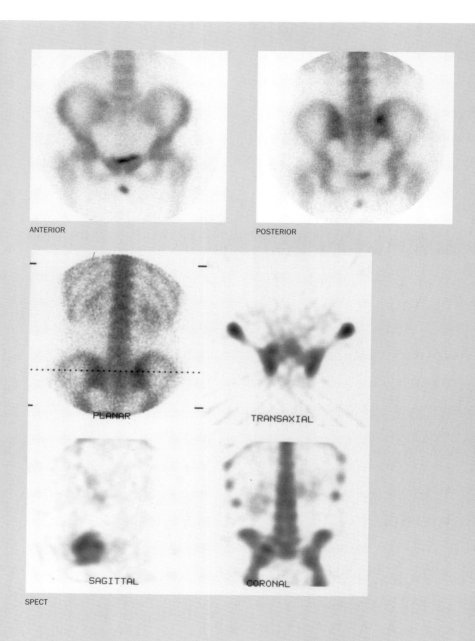

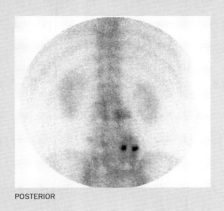

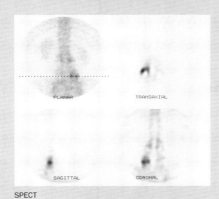

POSTERIOR   SPECT

Figure 7.23 Right pseudarthrosis in the lumbar fusion mass. This is the term given to an ununited fracture through the mass of new bone. Note also the uptake at the superior end of the fusion, due to arthritis. This commonly occurs at the extremities of a spinal fusion.

Disc pathology

The bone scan has no ability to demonstrate acute or chronic disc protrusion. Disc degeneration usually causes mild endplate uptake. Discitis can be diagnosed in its early phases by bone scanning. Gallium scanning is often used in conjunction. The classic sign of discitis on a bone scan is the presence of increased uptake of isotope in two adjacent vertebrae. As the degree of vertebral body involvement increases, vertebral osteomyelitis becomes more likely. Bone scans have been shown to be negative in some cases of discitis. A gallium scan is more sensitive in the detection of discitis prior to the complicating osteomyelitis (Fig. 7.24).

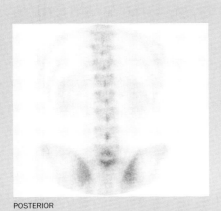

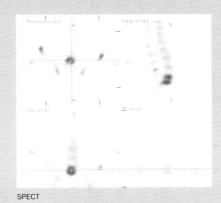

POSTERIOR   SPECT

Figure 7.24 L5/S1 discitis. Planar and SPECT images show increased uptake in the L5 and S1 vertebrae. This pattern of uptake in two adjacent vertebrae should raise the suspicion of discitis.

Other conditions

The bone scan shows no changes in Schmorl's nodes and Scheuermann's disease.

It is important to remember that many conditions such as an osteoid osteoma (Fig. 7.25), metastases, lymphoma, osteomyelitis and other benign and malignant conditions may cause bone pain that has been incorrectly attributed to sports injury. These conditions may be well demonstrated on bone scan.

Figure 7.25 An osteoid osteoma was an unexpected finding as a cause of back pain in an Olympic athlete.

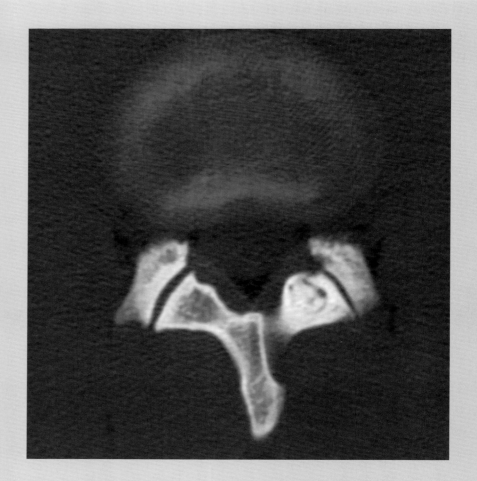

Bibliography

Bellah, RD, Summerville, DA, Treves, ST, Micheli, LJ, Low back pain in adolescent athletes: detection of stress injury to the pars interarticularis with SPECT, *Radiology* 180: 1991, pp 509–12

Choong, K, Monaghan, P, McGuigan, L, McLean, R, Role of bone scintigraphy in the early diagnosis of discitis, *Ann Rheum Dis* 49: 1990, pp 932–4

Collier, BD, Fogelman, I, Brown, ML, Bone scintigraphy: Part 2. Orthopedic bone scanning, *J Nucl Med* 34: 1993, pp 2241–6

Collier, BD, Hellman, RS, Krasnow, AZ, Bone SPECT, *Semin Nucl Med* 17: 1987, pp 247–66

Collier, BD, Johnson, RP, Carrera, GF, Meyer, GA, Schwab, JP, Flatley, TJ, Isitman, AT, Hellman, RS, Zielonka, JS, Knobel, J, Painful spondylolysis or spondylolisthesis studied by radiography and single-photon emission computed tomography, *Radiology* 154: 1985, pp 207–11

Even-Sapir, E, Martin, RH, Mitchell, MJ, et al., Assessment of painful late effects of lumbar fusion with SPECT, *J Nucl Med* 35: 1994, pp 416–22

Gates, GF, Oblique angle bone SPECT imaging of the lumbar spine, pelvis and hips. An anatomic study, *Clin Nucl Med* 21: 1996, pp 359–62

Gates, GF, Bone SPECT imaging of the painful back, *Clin Nucl Med* 21: 1996, pp 560–71

Gates, GF, SPECT bone scanning of the spine, *Semin Nucl Med* 28: 1998, pp 78–94

Holder, LE, Machin, JL, Asdourian, PL, Links, JM, Sexton, CC, Planar and high resolution SPECT bone imaging in the diagnosis of facet syndrome, *J Nucl Med* 36: 1995, pp 37–44

Kanmaz, B, Collier, BD, Liu, Y, Uzum, F, Uygur, G, Akansel, G, Gunes, I, Krasnow, AZ, Hellman, RS, Isitman, AT, Carrera, G, SPECT and three-phase planar bone scintigraphy in adults with chronic low back pain, *Nuclear Med Comm* 19: 1998, pp 13–21

Lowe, J, Schachner, E, Hirschberg, E, Shapiro, Y, Libson, E, Significance of bone scintigraphy in symptomatic spondylolysis, *Spine* 9: 1984, pp 653–5

Murray, IPC, Dixon, J, The role of single photon emission computed tomography in bone scintigraphy, *Skeletal Radiol* 18: 1989, pp 493–505

Pennell, RG, Maurer, AH, Bonakdarpour, A, Stress injuries of the pars interarticularis: radiographic classification and indications for scintigraphy, *AJR* 145: 1985, pp 763–6

Resnick, D, Nurayama, G, *Diagnosis of Bone & Joint Disorders*, WB Saunders Co., Philadelphia 1988, pp 1539–45

Slizofski, WJ, Collier, BD, Flatley, TJ, Carrera, GF, Hellman, RS, Isitman, AT, Painful pseudarthrosis following lumbar spinal fusion: detection by SPECT and planar scintigraphy, *Skel Radiol* 16: 1987, pp 136–41

Swanson, D, Blecker, I, Gahbauer, H, Caride, VJ, Diagnosis of discitis by SPECT technetium-99M MDP scintigram, *Clin Nucl Med* 12: 1987, pp 210–11.

Wiltse, LL, Widell, EH, Jackson, DW, Fatigue fracture: The basic lesion in isthmic spondylolisthesis, *J Bone and Joint Surg* [Am] 57: 1975, pp 17–22

8 The shoulder girdle and thorax

Almost all shoulder problems occurring as a result of sport are related to either instability or impingement. This means that the changes to be imaged are largely soft tissue and consequently the use of bone scans is limited. Although ultrasound and MRI play a major role, there are occasions when a bone scan may be helpful. The main advantage of bone scan is the wide coverage possible and if the symptoms are referred from changes in the cervical spine or thorax, these distant changes will be demonstrated. Bone scans are also useful for detecting occult fractures and bone stress around the shoulder girdle and thorax. The sternoclavicular joints can be particularly difficult to examine with plain films and, even with CT, subtle changes are often difficult to interpret. Rib fractures are also well demonstrated.

Tips on technique

Three-phase imaging is performed. For the flow study and blood pool images, the patient is placed with the point of clinical interest optimally positioned to view the part without superimposition of other structures. An anterior oblique view is usually used. The patient is supine, their arm by the side and the camera obliqued at approximately 30 degrees. The isotope is injected into the contralateral arm (or into a leg vein). Blood pool views of the opposite shoulder should also be obtained for comparison with the shoulders symmetrically positioned. If the field of view of the camera is large enough, an anterior view of both shoulders will allow simultaneous comparison.

The delayed images are usually obtained in the anterior and posterior oblique positions, again with 30 degrees camera angulation providing good separation of structures. Using the same degree of obliquity as a routine helps in scan interpretation. As Clunie et al. (1997) reported, the posterior oblique image provides the best separation of the humeral head from the glenoid and helps localisation. Images of the adjacent ribs and scapulae are obtained in these views. If abnormal uptake is seen in this region, repeat views with the arms elevated will change the position of the scapulae relative to the ribs. This will allow the uptake to be localised to either the scapula or underlying ribs. In addition, views of the sternum and sternoclavicular joints are obtained in the anterior projection. Cervical and thoracic spine views are obtained in the posterior projection, optimally with the neck and spine flexed against the camera head. The full length of the humeri and elbows are included in the study (Fig. 8.1).

Figure 8.1 Normal planar images of the shoulders and ribs. Note that the best image of the shoulder joint to separate the glenoid from the head of the humerus is the posterior oblique image. With many single head cameras both shoulders may not be imaged simultaneously in the anterior and posterior projections. Lateral views of the ribs may sometimes be added.

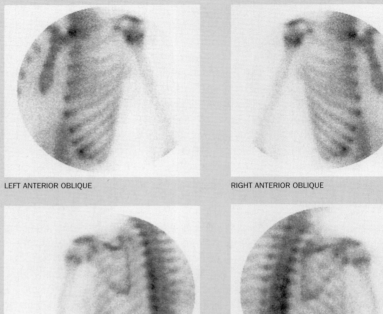

LEFT ANTERIOR OBLIQUE   RIGHT ANTERIOR OBLIQUE

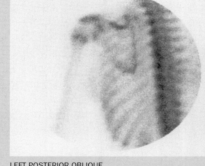
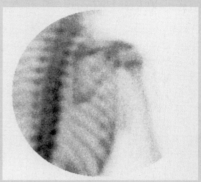

POSTERIOR   LEFT POSTERIOR OBLIQUE   RIGHT POSTERIOR OBLIQUE

Fractures (Figs 8.2–8.13)

A bone scan is useful for demonstrating occult fractures, bone stress and stress fractures. Fractures of the ribs and sternum are very common and many of these fractures are difficult to detect on plain films. Scapular fractures are less common but are equally difficult to appreciate on plain films. In practical terms, when symptoms persist, a negative scan excludes recent fracture.

Figure 8.2 Fracture of the right fourth rib. The second image with the arm elevated and the patient in an oblique position demonstrates that the abnormality is definitely in rib and not in scapula. The fracture has a more linear appearance than usual.

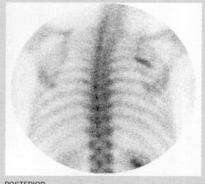
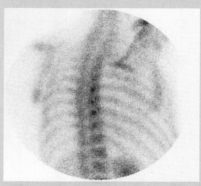

POSTERIOR   RIGHT POSTERIOR OBLIQUE

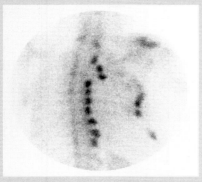

RIGHT POSTERIOR OBLIQUE

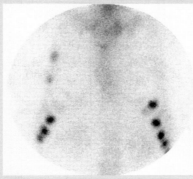

ANTERIOR

Figure 8.3 Three separate cases of multiple rib fractures due to direct trauma. In all cases the preceding X-rays were normal. In the first case there was also evidence of a fracture in the scapula close to the glenoid.

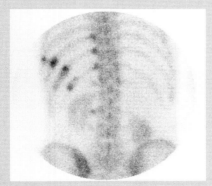

POSTERIOR

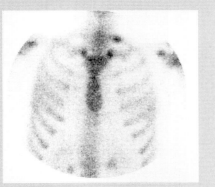

ANTERIOR

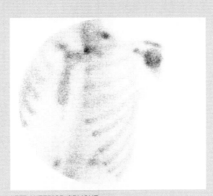

LEFT ANTERIOR OBLIQUE

Figure 8.4 Fracture of the left first rib posteriorly.

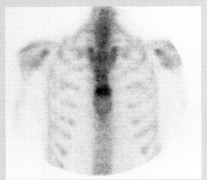

ANTERIOR

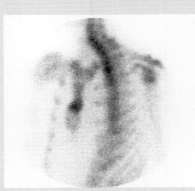

LEFT ANTERIOR OBLIQUE

Figure 8.5 Transverse fracture in the mid sternum.

Figure 8.6 Oblique fracture of the body of the sternum.

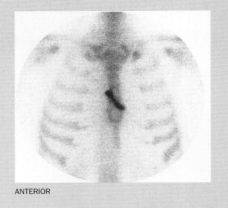

ANTERIOR

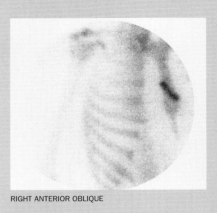

RIGHT ANTERIOR OBLIQUE

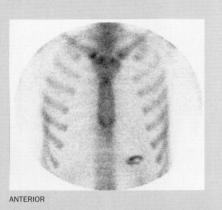

ANTERIOR

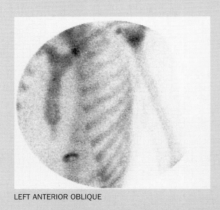

LEFT ANTERIOR OBLIQUE

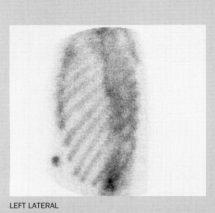

LEFT LATERAL

Figure 8.7 Calcification in a torn left costal cartilage. There is no abnormal uptake in bone.

Figure 8.8 Trauma to the right first chondrosternal junction. The oblique images help differentiate the post-traumatic calcification of the costal cartilage from the more common sternoclavicular joint arthritis.

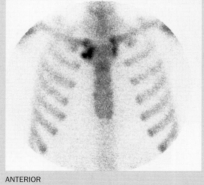

ANTERIOR

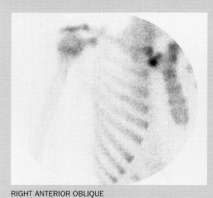

RIGHT ANTERIOR OBLIQUE

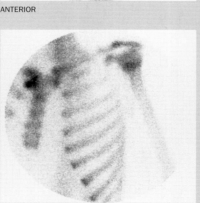

LEFT ANTERIOR OBLIQUE

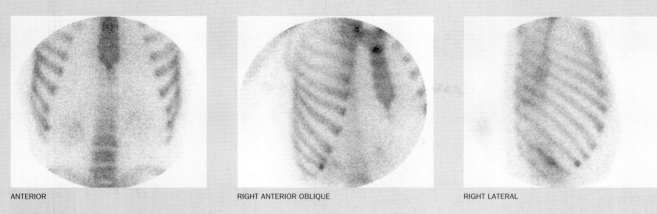

ANTERIOR   RIGHT ANTERIOR OBLIQUE   RIGHT LATERAL

Figure 8.9 Right tenth costochondral junction injury due to direct trauma. There is focal low-grade uptake in the costochondral junction, best seen in the lateral projection.

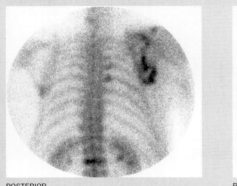
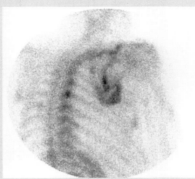
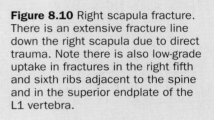

POSTERIOR   RIGHT POSTERIOR OBLIQUE

Figure 8.10 Right scapula fracture. There is an extensive fracture line down the right scapula due to direct trauma. Note there is also low-grade uptake in fractures in the right fifth and sixth ribs adjacent to the spine and in the superior endplate of the L1 vertebra.

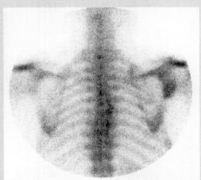
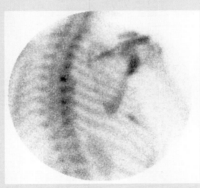
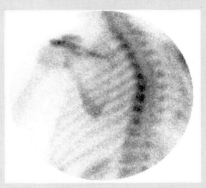

POSTERIOR   RIGHT POSTERIOR OBLIQUE   LEFT POSTERIOR OBLIQUE

Figure 8.11 Fracture of the right scapula close to the glenoid. There is also a fracture in the right seventh rib. Both of these injuries were due to a fall on the right side. The left posterior oblique view is included for comparison.

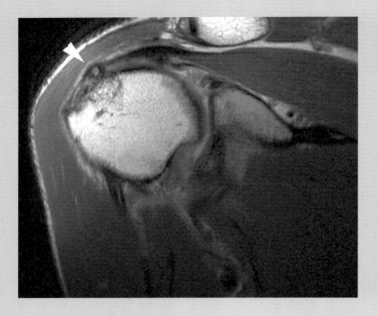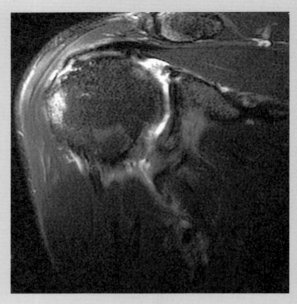

Figure 8.12 Following trauma there has been avulsion of a small fragment from the insertion of the supraspinatus tendon with retraction. The T1 weighted image shows the retracted fragment (arrow) and, in the T2 weighted image, extensive high signal is seen associated with the fracture. Deformity of the superior labrum is typical of a SLAP lesion.

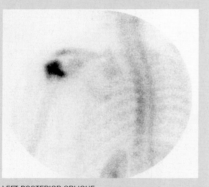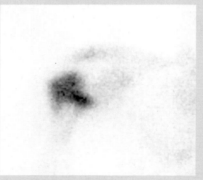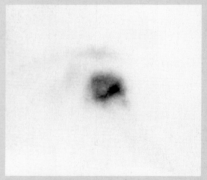

LEFT POSTERIOR OBLIQUE   ZOOM LEFT POSTERIOR OBLIQUE   ZOOM LEFT ANTERIOR OBLIQUE

Figure 8.13 Comminuted fracture of the left humeral head with an avascular fragment posteromedially. This was due to a direct fall onto the shoulder. The intensity of the magnified images is adjusted to show the fracture detail.

Stress fractures around the shoulder girdle are unusual but have been described in baseball, weightlifting, racquet sports, diving and trapshooting. Stress fractures in the ribs have been described in rowers, golfers, dancers, scuba divers, archers and baseball pitchers. While focal uptake is the commonest appearance, linear uptake along the rib may also be seen, and it can be difficult to determine if this is due to a linear fracture or to periostitis (Figs 8.14–8.16).

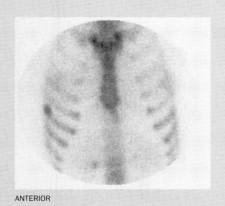 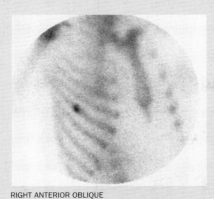

Figure 8.14 Stress fracture in the right seventh rib laterally in a rower.

ANTERIOR

RIGHT ANTERIOR OBLIQUE

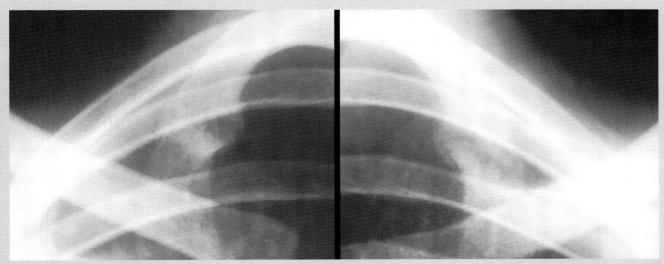

BILATERAL STRESS FRACTURES OF THE FIRST RIBS OF A MALE DANCER.

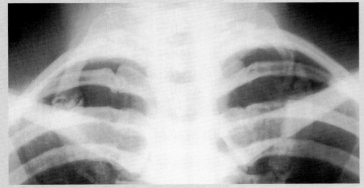

BILATERAL STRESS FRACTURES OF THE FIRST RIBS OF A SCUBA DIVER.

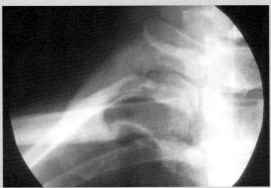

A STRESS FRACTURE OF A FIRST RIB OF A BASEBALL PITCHER.

Figure 8.15 Stress fractures in ribs

Figure 8.16 Linear uptake in the left eleventh rib in a cricket fast bowler. This abnormal uptake indicates stress reaction, probably due to periosteal traction injury. The prominent uptake at the left scapular tip on the left posterior oblique view is due to summation effect as the scapula tip overlies the rib.

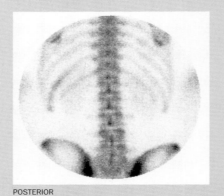

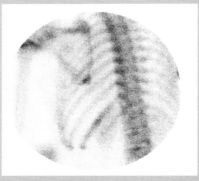

POSTERIOR

LEFT POSTERIOR OBLIQUE

Enthesopathies (Figs 8.17–8.22)

Enthesopathies around the shoulder characteristically result from repetitive movements and often present as poorly localised symptoms. A bone scan will define the site of the problem. A common enthesopathy seen in the shoulder occurs at the supraspinatus tendon insertion. This is detected as a small focus of increased uptake in the superolateral portion of the humeral head, seen on the delayed views. Other enthesopathies occur in the proximal shaft of the humerus medially. It is often difficult to determine exactly which muscle insertion is involved and further clarification can be obtained with MRI.

Scapular enthesopathies can be seen at the medial and lateral borders inferiorly and in the spine of the scapula. Coracoid uptake is variable, making it difficult to diagnose an enthesopathy at the short head of biceps/coracobrachialis origin.

Figure 8.17 Right supraspinatus enthesopathy in the right humeral head. Note that the localised focus of uptake at the supraspinatus insertion site differentiates this condition from the more diffuse uptake in glenohumeral arthritis.

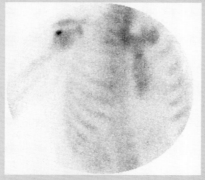

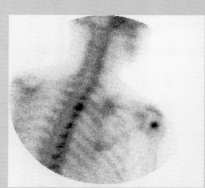

RIGHT ANTERIOR OBLIQUE

RIGHT POSTERIOR OBLIQUE

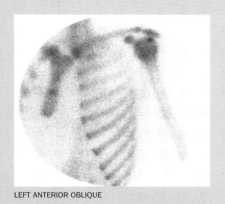

LEFT ANTERIOR OBLIQUE

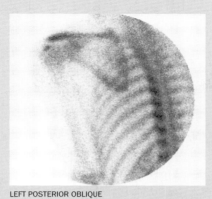

LEFT POSTERIOR OBLIQUE

Figure 8.18 Low-grade left supraspinatus enthesopathy.

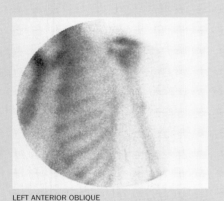

LEFT ANTERIOR OBLIQUE

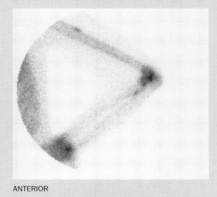

ANTERIOR

Figure 8.19 Enthesopathy at the left deltoid insertion in the humerus. Note that there is also a low-grade enthesopathy in the radial tuberosity at the biceps insertion.

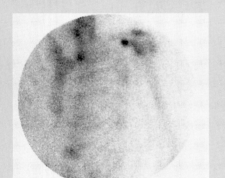
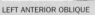

LEFT ANTERIOR OBLIQUE

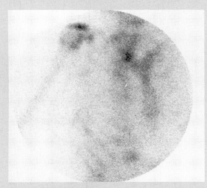

RIGHT ANTERIOR OBLIQUE

Figure 8.20 Left coracoid enthesopathy. Several muscles arise at this site and may give rise to the enthesopathy. The intensity of coracoid uptake is very variable and pathology should be diagnosed on the scan only when there is significant asymmetry.

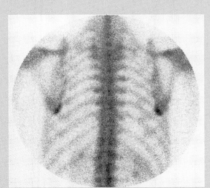

POSTERIOR

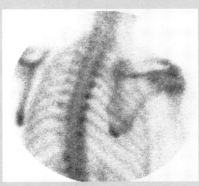

RIGHT POSTERIOR OBLIQUE

Figure 8.21 Serratus anterior enthesopathies at the tips of the scapulae. There is focal increase in uptake in the tips of both scapulae, with the oblique view demonstrating that this is not due to a summation artefact. This occurred in a man who had recently undertaken a sudden increase in weight training.

Figure 8.22 Low-grade enthesopathy at the lateral border of the right scapula. The oblique and arms-up views demonstrate that the focus is in the scapula rather than the rib. This abnormality was due to repetitive throwing.

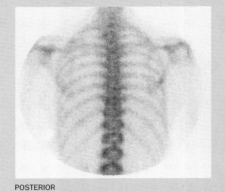

POSTERIOR

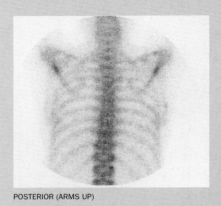

POSTERIOR (ARMS UP)

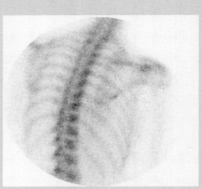

RIGHT POSTERIOR OBLIQUE

Arthritis/frozen shoulder (Fig. 8.23)

Degenerative changes in the glenohumeral joint are relatively uncommon and usually result from trauma that has involved the articular surfaces. Degenerative arthritis is well demonstrated on bone scan. Adhesive capsulitis or frozen shoulder is commonly seen in older patients after injury. The bone scan appearance is of intense uptake throughout the joint.

Figure 8.23 Right acromioclavicular joint arthritis. There is increased uptake of isotope in both sides of the right acromioclavicular joint with relatively normal uptake in the glenohumeral joint. This is a common scan finding, especially in the post-traumatic setting.

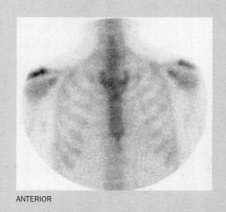

ANTERIOR

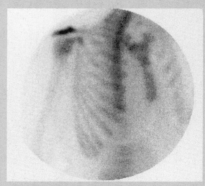

RIGHT ANTERIOR OBLIQUE

Muscle injury (Figs 8.24–8.26)

Quite early after muscle injury, a diffusely increased uptake may be seen. The uptake may also be seen in a specific muscle or muscle group following overuse such as may occur in weight training. Myositis ossificans produces an intense uptake in the active phase.

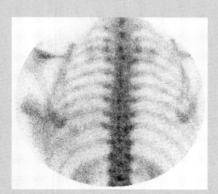

POSTERIOR

Figure 8.24 Left latissimus dorsi muscle acute tear. The abnormal uptake is confined to soft tissue.

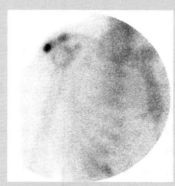

RIGHT ANTERIOR OBLIQUE

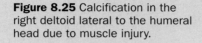

RIGHT POSTERIOR OBLIQUE

Figure 8.25 Calcification in the right deltoid lateral to the humeral head due to muscle injury.

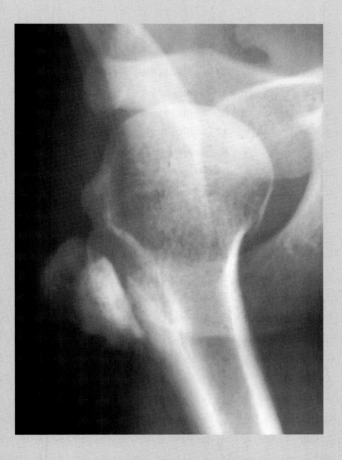

Figure 8.26 Myositis ossificans has developed adjacent to the bicipital groove following an avulsion injury at the pectoralis major insertion.

Other conditions (Figs 8.27 and 8.28)

Non-sports causes of shoulder girdle pain should also be considered.

Figure 8.27 Marrow invasion secondary to leukaemia. Note the irregular uptake in the left humeral shaft and sternum with reduced uptake in the upper portion of the body of the sternum. The rib uptake is relatively high and slightly uneven. Similar diffuse increase and uneven uptake were seen in the rest of the skeleton and proximal long bones. This patient presented with shoulder pain from a sports clinic.

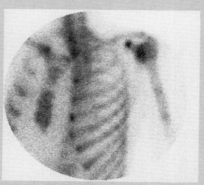

LEFT ANTERIOR OBLIQUE

Figure 8.28 Right axillary vein thrombosis. The initial injection through the left antecubital fossa to assess right shoulder pain showed relatively normal flow and blood pool images of the right arm (top row). The delayed bone images (not shown) also appeared normal. Because of swelling in the right arm and the absence of bony pathology, a second injection into the right antecubital fossa was performed and the second flow and blood pool images revealed the axillary vein thrombosis and collateral flow (bottom row).

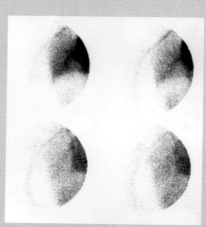

FLOW RIGHT ANTERIOR OBLIQUE

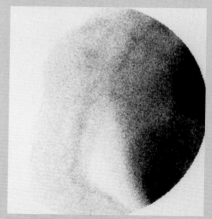

BLOOD POOL RIGHT ANTERIOR OBLIQUE

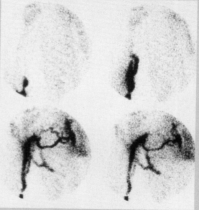

FLOW RIGHT ANTERIOR OBLIQUE

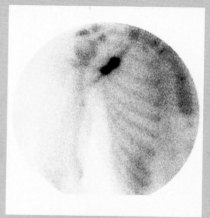

BLOOD POOL RIGHT ANTERIOR OBLIQUE

Bibliography

Clunie, G, Bomanji, J, Ell, PJ, Tc 99m-MDP patterns in patients with painful shoulder lesions, *J Nucl Med* 38: 1997, pp 1491–5

Hall, RJ, Calvert, PT, Stress fracture of the acromion: an unusual mechanism & review of the literature, *J Bone Joint Surg* [Br] 77: 1995, pp 153–4

Horwitz, BR, Di Stefano, V, Stress fracture of the humerus in a weightlifter, *Orthopedics* 18: 1995, pp 185–7

Patel, M, Upper extremity radionuclide bone imaging: Shoulder, arm, elbow, and forearm, *Semin Nucl Med* 28: 1998, pp 3–13.

Schils, JP, Freed, HA, Richmond, BJ, Piraino, DW, Bergfeld, JA, Belhobek, GH, Stress fracture of the acromion, *Am J Roentgenol* 155: 1990, pp 1140–1

9 The elbow and forearm

The elbow is anatomically exposed and acute injuries often occur as the result of direct trauma or indirectly from a fall onto the hand and wrist. The throwing action may cause both acute and overuse injury due to valgus stress and hyperextension. Twisting and hyperextension injuries contribute to acute trauma. Repetitive stress occurring at the extensor and flexor origins is also a common cause of elbow problems.

The role of nuclear medicine in imaging sporting injuries at the elbow joint is limited. The elbow is a difficult joint to image on bone scan and the resulting images may be difficult to interpret. This is especially so in the young when uptake of isotope in the multiple growth plates can obscure pathological changes. Fractures and enthesopathies are the injuries most commonly requiring bone scan.

Tips on technique

Attention to optimal positioning is critical and as in other areas it is important to obtain images in orthogonal planes (Fig. 9.1).

Good visualisation of the medial and lateral epicondyles of the elbow is achieved with the hands supinated and the elbows resting on the collimator face (posterior view). Taping the hands helps the patient remain still and avoids a slow creep out of supination. It is important that the head doesn't become superimposed over the elbows. A skyline or tangential view with the elbow flexed is also used for showing the epicondyles. Although this is easier for the patient, superimposition prevents examination of the remainder of the elbow.

For imaging the forearm bones, medial elbow and olecranon region, images with the elbows flexed and the forearms resting on the collimator face (medial view) generally give the best results. Lateral elbows views can be obtained with the camera face vertical and the patient seated with their hand on their hip or with the patient supine, elbow flexed, arm abducted and with the lateral aspect of the elbow resting against the collimator.

It is important not to inject the cubital fossa of either the elbow of interest or the opposite side. The opposite hand or a leg vein should be used. The technologist should record the injection site.

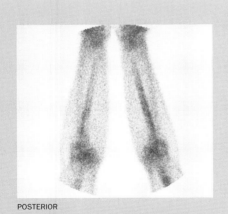
POSTERIOR

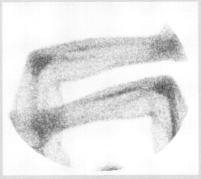

MEDIALS

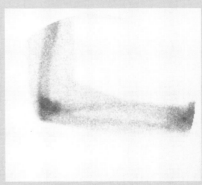
RIGHT LATERAL

Figure 9.1 Standard views.

Fractures (Figs 9.2–9.6)

If initial plain films are normal but a high index of suspicion of fracture persists, a bone scan is indicated to help exclude an occult fracture. A persisting elbow effusion on plain films is also a sign suggestive of an occult fracture. As with fractures elsewhere, the typical appearance is of a focal increase uptake of isotope on the blood pool images and increased uptake on the delayed images.

Of all fractures at the elbow, a radial head or neck fracture is the fracture causing the greatest diagnostic problem. This fracture may be difficult to diagnose confidently on plain films and a bone scan can be necessary to establish or confirm a diagnosis. Occasionally this fracture is seen as an unexpected incidental finding. In the immature elbow, the fracture can involve the epiphysis or growth plate. Stress fractures of the radial head and neck also occur and can result from repetitive compression forces in the lateral joint space usually produced by the throwing action. These lateral compressive forces are secondary to traction on the medial side that can cause ligamentous injury to the medial collateral ligament or an avulsion at the medial epicondyle or medial corner of the coronoid. In the immature elbow, avulsion of the medial epicondylar apophysis may occur.

Figure 9.2 Bilateral radial head fractures. The uptake in both radial heads flares into the adjacent shaft of the radius. There is an associated low-grade fracture in the left hamate. The injury occurred due to a fall from a horse.

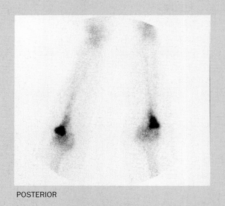

POSTERIOR

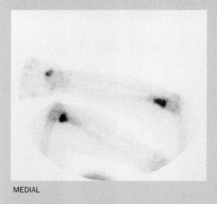

MEDIAL

Figure 9.3 Fracture of the left radial head associated with a fracture of the left scaphoid. This is a common association and the radial head fracture may be relatively asymptomatic compared to the scaphoid fracture. Imaging for a wrist injury should always include imaging of the forearms and elbows.

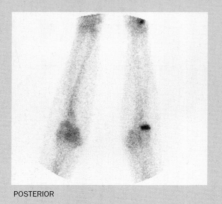

POSTERIOR

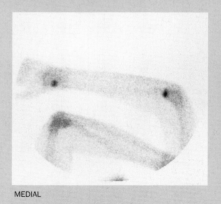

MEDIAL

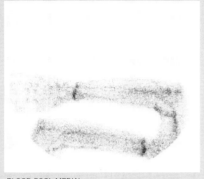

BLOOD POOL MEDIAL

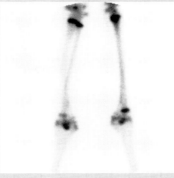

POSTERIOR

Figure 9.4 Fracture through the left radial head growth plate in a child. The increase in vascularity and asymmetry on the blood pool image is a helpful sign in diagnosing growth plate fracture in children. Note that the many normal growth plates in the elbows make fracture detection in children more difficult. Any growth plate asymmetry in a well-positioned image should be viewed with suspicion.

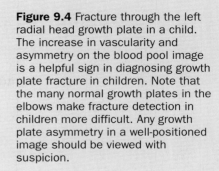

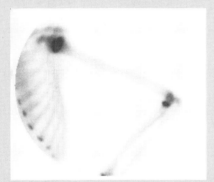

LEFT LATERAL

Figure 9.5 A stress fracture of the radial neck of an adolescent tennis player, resulting from compressive forces in the lateral side of the elbow joint associated with racquet sports.

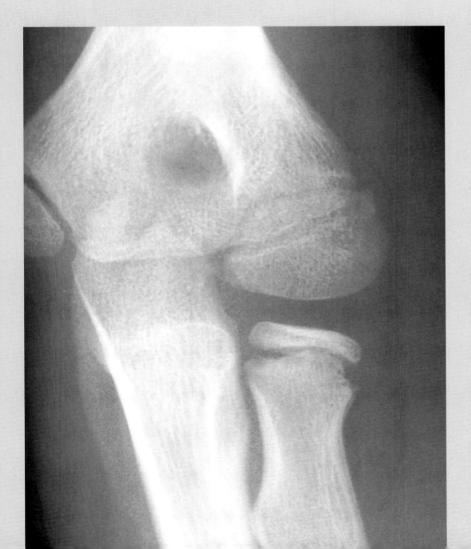

Figure 9.6 Fracture of the proximal left radius. The uptake on both the blood pool and the delayed images is maximal at the radial tuberosity but flares along the radius in both directions. The fact that the uptake extends across the bone distinguishes fracture from the common enthesopathy at this site. Traumatic synovitis is also present in the elbow.

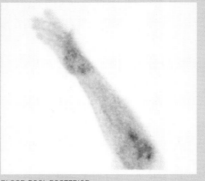

BLOOD POOL POSTERIOR

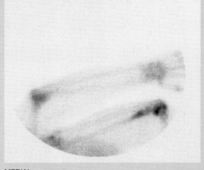

MEDIAL

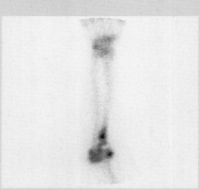

POSTERIOR

A supracondylar fracture of the humerus is the commonest elbow fracture seen in the immature athlete. Fractures of the olecranon usually result from a fall on the tip of the elbow or triceps avulsion, and fractures of the coronoid process are usually the legacy of a dislocation. Bone scans are required only occasionally for the diagnosis of these elbow fractures.

Similarly, simple forearm fractures usually do not require a bone scan for diagnosis. However, plastic bowing of the forearm bones can occur. This condition produces a characteristic bone-scan pattern, with a diffuse increase in uptake occurring along the entire shaft of the forearm bone involved.

Bone stress involving the forearm is uncommon. However the authors have seen two cases in the midshaft of the ulna in elite tennis players. Interestingly, the stress changes are on the non-dominant side and result from the double-handed backhand. This bone stress has also been described in softball pitchers and is thought to result from torsion (Figs 9.7–9.13).

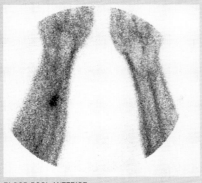

BLOOD POOL ANTERIOR

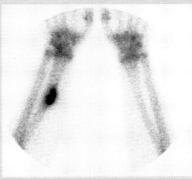

ANTERIOR

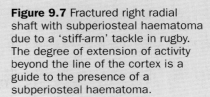

Figure 9.7 Fractured right radial shaft with subperiosteal haematoma due to a 'stiff-arm' tackle in rugby. The degree of extension of activity beyond the line of the cortex is a guide to the presence of a subperiosteal haematoma.

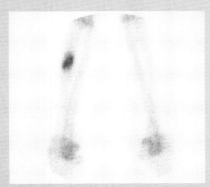

POSTERIOR

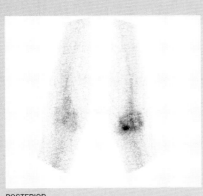

POSTERIOR

MEDIAL

Figure 9.8 Fracture of the left olecranon tip at its medial edge due to direct trauma. There is associated traumatic synovitis in the elbow joint.

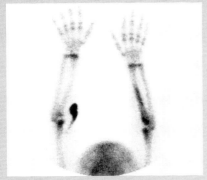

ANTERIOR (PALMAR)

Figure 9.9 Fracture of the proximal left radial shaft in a child. Fractures in the long bones in young children may show diffuse uptake along the shaft rather than a discrete focus. Plastic deformity may be associated with this.

Figure 9.10 Plastic deformity fractures in right ulna and radius. This unusual injury occurred when the adolescent patient had his arm caught in an industrial roller.

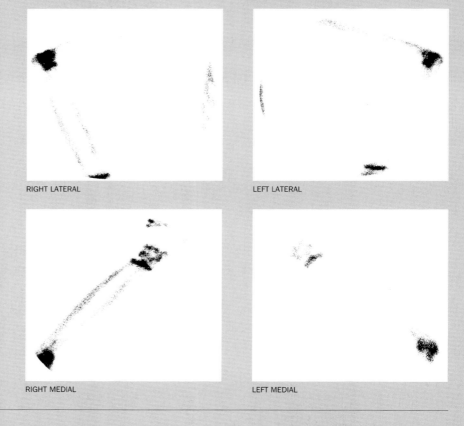

RIGHT LATERAL

LEFT LATERAL

RIGHT MEDIAL

LEFT MEDIAL

Figure 9.11 Stress fracture in the midshaft of the left ulna in a left-handed elite tennis player.

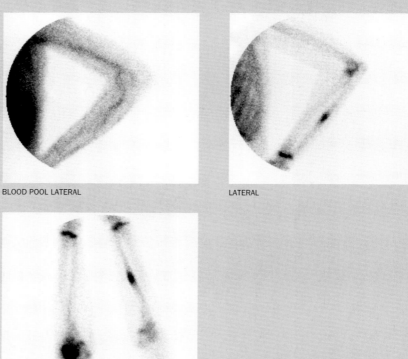

BLOOD POOL LATERAL

LATERAL

POSTERIOR

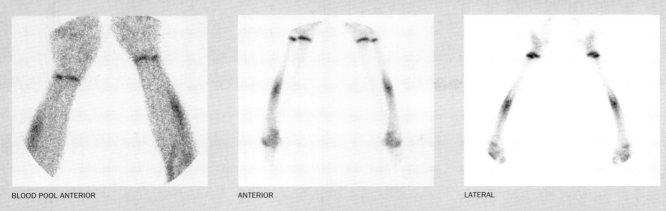

BLOOD POOL ANTERIOR   ANTERIOR   LATERAL

Figure 9.12 Bilateral ulnar shaft stress fractures secondary to weight training. Note there is focal activity with flaring along both shafts on both the blood pool and the delayed images.

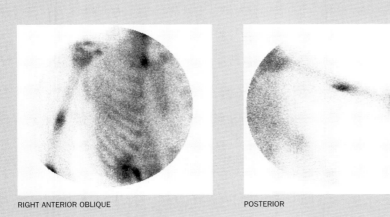

RIGHT ANTERIOR OBLIQUE   POSTERIOR

Figure 9.13 Stress fracture in the right humeral shaft.

Enthesopathies (Figs 9.14–9.18)

Ultrasound is the imaging modality of choice in the evaluation of tendon and muscle pathology around the elbow joint. However the bone scan is extremely sensitive in the detection of abnormalities at the tendon/bone interface. The early blood pool images are usually normal. The delayed views show a focus of uptake at the site of ligament or tendon insertion.

Lateral epicondylitis ('tennis elbow') is the commonest enthesopathy around the elbow and usually results from overuse related to excessive wrist extension. As this condition is so common, changes at the epicondyle may also be seen as an incidental finding.

Medial epicondylitis ('golfer's elbow') results from excessive throwing activity, golf or forehand tennis strokes. Both lateral and medial epicondylitis are best imaged using the posterior view. The medial or lateral views may help confirm the site of pathology.

Figure 9.14 Left lateral epicondylitis. There is focal increase in uptake over the left lateral epicondyle, seen best on the posterior elbow view with the elbows extended. Imaging in two planes is always required for accurate localisation. The right lateral view is included for comparison.

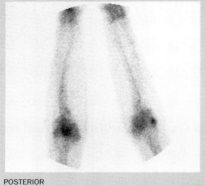

POSTERIOR

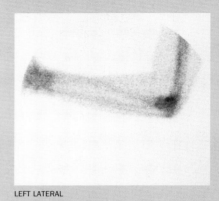

LEFT LATERAL

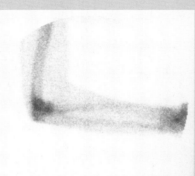

RIGHT LATERAL

Figure 9.15 Bilateral lateral epicondylitis, more marked on the right.

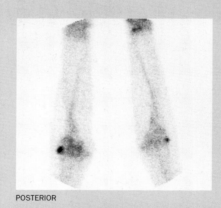

POSTERIOR

Figure 9.16 Left medial epicondylitis.

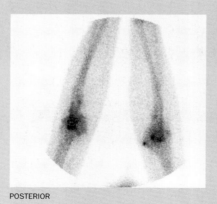

POSTERIOR

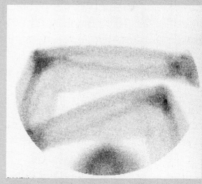

MEDIAL

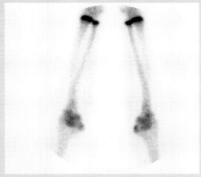

POSTERIOR

Figure 9.17 Traction injury to the left medial epicondyle growth plate. In children, the growth plate represents a relatively weak region of the bone and is at greater risk of fracture or traction injury. This case also demonstrates the difficulty in interpreting bone scans of the elbows in children due to the multiple growth plates. Careful attention to symmetrical positioning is essential.

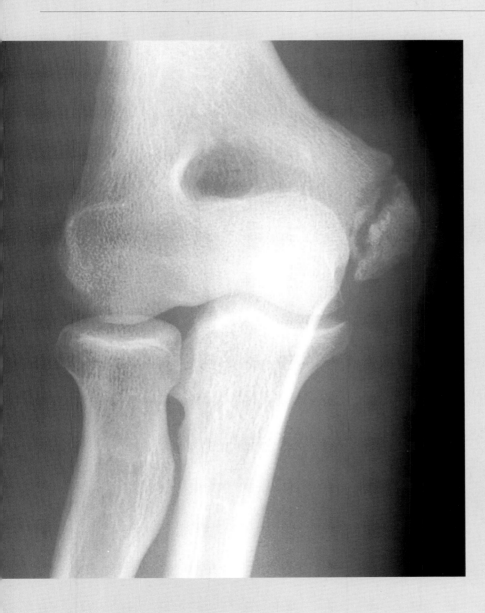

Figure 9.18 Avulsion of the medial epicondylar apophysis in an immature athlete due to medial traction forces.

Triceps enthesopathy is best seen on the medial view. This position reduces the tendency to move and the camera is closer to the olecranon. The typical appearance is of increased uptake at the triceps insertion (Figs 9.19–9.21).

Figure 9.19 Enthesopathies at the insertion of the triceps tendons, more marked in the left olecranon. The blood pool image (not shown) was normal. There is a small focus of increased uptake on the delayed images at the insertion sites. Mild bilateral medial epicondylitis is also present.

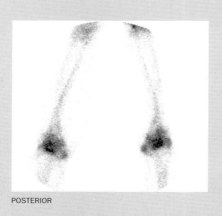
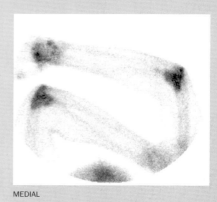

POSTERIOR   MEDIAL

Figure 9.20 Repetitive triceps traction resulting in an olecranon avulsion.

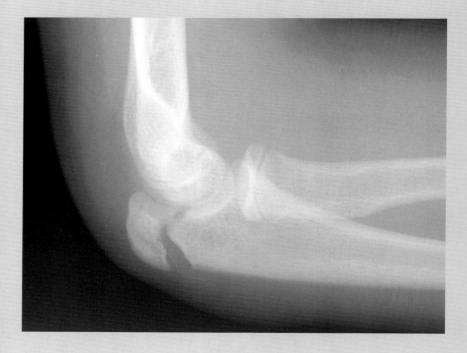

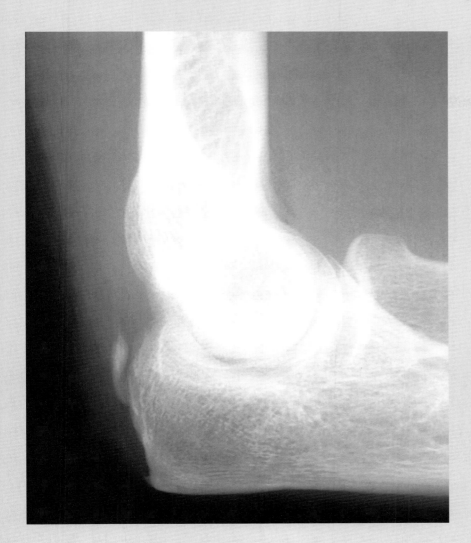

Figure 9.21 Calcific tendinopathy of the triceps.

Another source of obscure pain in the elbow region is an enthesopathy at the biceps brachii insertion at the radial tuberosity. Focal uptake is seen on both the posterior and medial views confined to the radial tuberosity. It may be difficult to distinguish this from the less common brachialis enthesopathy at the ulnar tuberosity. Care should be taken with correct positioning, particularly in the posterior view, making sure the arms are symmetrically supinated to the greatest practical degree. The ulnar tuberosity is then more medial than the radial tuberosity (Figs 9.22 and 9.23).

Figure 9.22 Left biceps enthesopathy at the radial tuberosity. Note that there is also uptake at the tip of the right olecranon due to olecranon impingement.

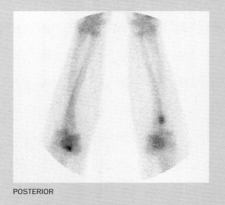

POSTERIOR

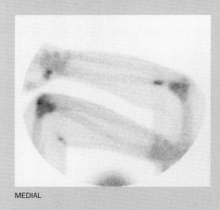

MEDIAL

Figure 9.23 Left brachialis enthesopathy at the ulnar tuberosity. This is much less common than biceps enthesopathy, the distinguishing feature being that the uptake is more medial on the posterior (supinated) images when the ulnar tuberosity is the site of pathology.

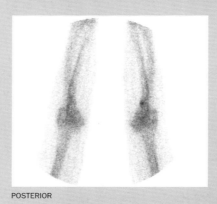

POSTERIOR

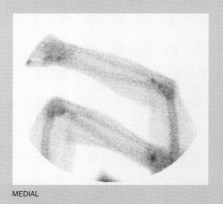

MEDIAL

Obscure pain above the elbow may arise from enthesopathy at the origin of the brachialis muscle, causing linear periosteal uptake in the distal humeral shaft anteriorly. The authors have seen this in volleyball and tennis players, associated with rapid rotation of the elbow during spiking and serving (Figs 9.24 and 9.25).

Figure 9.24 Enthesopathy at the brachialis origin in the distal right humerus of a tennis player. Note that the uptake is in a linear periosteal distribution. The term 'arm splints' has been used for this condition.

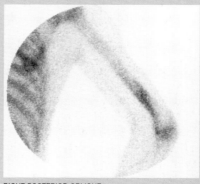

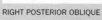

RIGHT POSTERIOR OBLIQUE

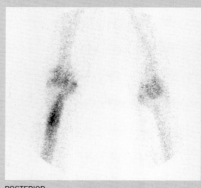

POSTERIOR

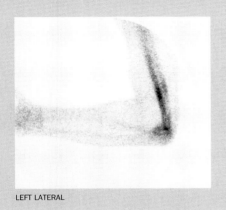

Figure 9.25 Left arm splint. There is an extensive enthesopathy at the origin of the brachialis.

LEFT LATERAL

'Ulnar splints' is a phenomenon due to repetitive weightbearing movements of the wrists as occurs in weight training (curls). It is akin to the periosteal reaction in the shins, presenting with poorly localised pain in the forearms. On the bone scan there is a linear increase in uptake in a periosteal distribution along the shaft of the ulna (Figs 9.26 and 9.27).

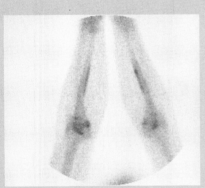

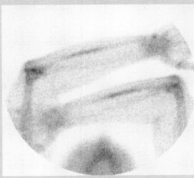

Figure 9.26 Bilateral ulnar 'splints'. There is linear periosteal uptake in the medial midshaft of the ulnae secondary to weight training (curls).

POSTERIOR

MEDIAL

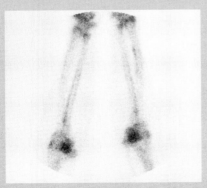

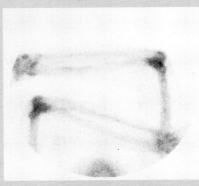

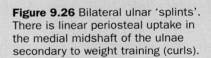

Figure 9.27 Bilateral ulnar and radial 'splints' secondary to weight training.

POSTERIOR

MEDIAL

Enthesopathy at the insertion of the ulnar collateral ligament on the coronoid process of the ulna results from ligament strain and should be distinguished from medial epicondylitis and focal arthritis (Fig. 9.28).

Figure 9.28 Bilateral coronoid process enthesopathies at the ulnar collateral ligament insertions, left more marked than the right. The uptake should not be confused with medial epicondylitis. The line of activity in the distal humeri is of uncertain aetiology.

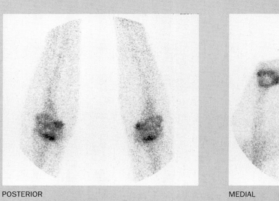

POSTERIOR

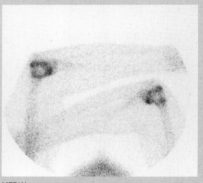

MEDIAL

Other conditions (Figs 9.29–9.35)

Olecranon impingement may result from repeated forced elbow hyper-extension. This has been well described in baseball players, fast bowlers and players in other throwing sports. Soft tissue and bony impingement occurs, producing posterior elbow pain. The bone scan shows a small focus of uptake at the posterior tip of the trochlear notch and/or in the olecranon fossa.

Olecranon bursitis should not be confused with triceps enthesopathy. The olecranon bursa is a subcutaneous structure and the diagnosis of bursitis is usually clinical. With bursitis, the bone scan generally shows a greater degree of soft tissue vascularity than in triceps enthesopathy and there is less bone uptake on the delayed views.

Arthritis in the elbow may be seen in the older athlete. However post-traumatic synovitis or premature osteoarthritis may occur in the younger age group. The bone scan shows increased uptake on the articular surfaces of the elbow. The uptake may be either diffuse or more focal, depending on the extent of involvement.

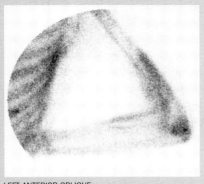

Figure 9.29 Bilateral muscle uptake in the distal humeri and proximal forearms due to an episode of excessive weight training.

LEFT ANTERIOR OBLIQUE

RIGHT ANTERIOR OBLIQUE

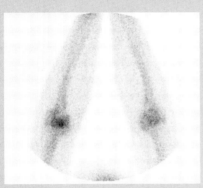
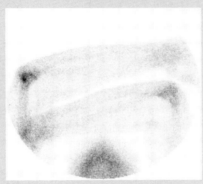

Figure 9.30 Right olecranon impingement. There is a focus of uptake in the olecranon fossa, indicating olecranon impingement. This can occur due to acute hyperextension or due to chronic impingement, particularly in throwing sports.

POSTERIOR

MEDIAL

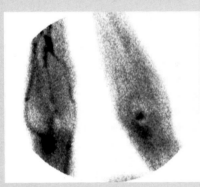

Figure 9.31 Left olecranon bursitis. The blood pool images show marked increase in vascularity superficially over the extensor surface of the left elbow with focal increase in the olecranon tip. Note that the patient was injected in the right hand to avoid confusion due to possible extravasation. The delayed images show focal increase in uptake at the olecranon tip, but no flaring into the body of the olecranon. This intensity of delayed uptake is more than is usually seen in this condition. The absence of flaring deeper into bone is evidence against osteomyelitis.

BLOOD POOL POSTERIOR

BLOOD POOL MEDIAL

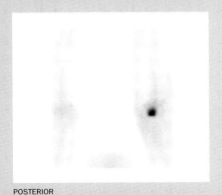

POSTERIOR

MEDIAL

Figure 9.32 A typical plain film appearance of olecranon bursitis.

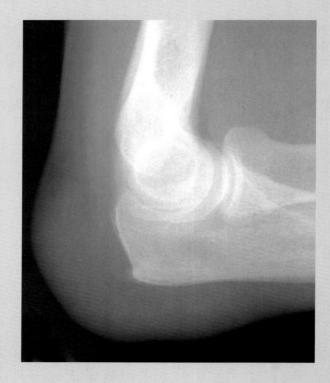

Figure 9.33 Left elbow arthritis affecting the entire joint.

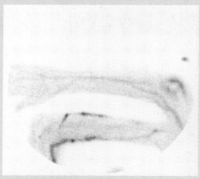

BLOOD POOL MEDIAL

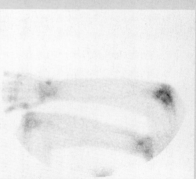

MEDIAL

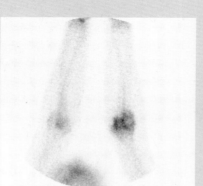

POSTERIOR

POSTERIOR

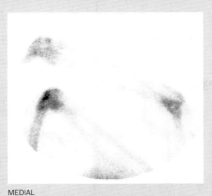

MEDIAL

Figure 9.34 Osteochondritis dissecans of the right capitellum. Olecranon impingement is also present. The low-grade focal uptake on the capitellum is not seen on the medial view because of super-imposed bone.

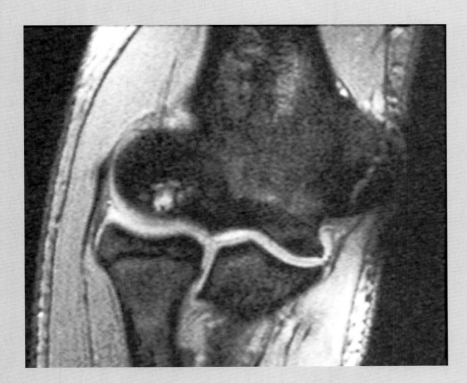

Figure 9.35 Developing osteo-chondritis dissecans of the capitellum demonstrated by a STIR MR image. There is high signal in the medulla and abnormal signal in the overlying articular cartilage.

Osteochondritis dissecans of the capitellum may occur with repetitive trauma at the radiocapitellar joint. It is difficult to diagnose on bone scan and MRI is the preferred method of imaging this process.

Bibliography

Bollen, SR, Robinson, DG, Crichton, KJ, Cross, MJ, Stress fractures of the ulna in tennis players using a double handed backhand stroke, *Am J Sports Med* 21: 1993, pp 751–2

Fink-Bennett, D, Carichner, S, Acute flexion of the elbow: Optimal imaging position for visualisation of the capitellum, *Clin Nucl Med* 11: 1986, pp 667–8

Gore, RM, Rogers, LF, Bowerman, J, Suker, J, Compere, CL, Osseous manifestations of elbow stress associated with sports activities, *AJR* 134: 1980, pp 971–7

Miller, JE, Javelin throwing elbow, *J Bone Joint Surg* 42: 1960, pp 788–92

Mutoh, Y, Mori, T, Suzuki, Y, Suzuira, Y, Stress fractures in the ulna in athletes, *Am J Sports Med* 10: 1982, pp 365–7

Patel, M, Upper extremity radionuclide bone imaging: shoulder, arm, elbow & forearm, *Semin Nucl Med* 28: 1998, pp 3–13

Plancker, KD, Halbrecht, J, Laurie, GM, Medial and lateral epicondylitis in the athlete, *Clinics in Sports Medicine* 15: 1996, pp 283–305

Rettig, AC, Stress fracture of the ulna in an adolescent tournament tennis player, *Am J Sports Med* 11: 1980, pp 103–6

Roach, PJ, Cooper, RA, Watson, AS, Arm splints seen on bone scan in a volleyball player, *Clin Nucl Med* 18: 1993, pp 900–1

Van Der Wall, H, Frater, CJ, Magee, MA, Kannangara, S, Bruce, W, Murray, IPC, A novel view for the scintigraphic assessment of the elbow, *Nucl Med Comm* 20: 1999, pp 1059–65

Woodward, AH, Bianco, AJ Jr, Osteochondritis dissecans of the elbow, *Clin Orthop* 110: 1975, pp 35–41

10 The hand and wrist

Imaging of the hand and wrist has become more precise as increased importance is placed on the early diagnosis and management of hand and wrist injuries. This change of attitude is the result of a better appreciation of the disabilities resulting from sporting injuries that are either ignored or inappropriately treated. There is also improved appreciation of the short time available for optimal surgical management of many tendon injuries, instabilities and fractures.

Plain films play a major role in the diagnosis of hand injuries, but the complexity of the anatomy of the wrist limits the effectiveness of plain films in the diagnosis of injury in this region. Both soft tissue and bone are injured following wrist trauma and all imaging modalities are used in wrist imaging. As a general rule symptoms on the ulnar side of the wrist are usually due to soft tissue injury, and radial pain and disability are produced more often from bone injury. Bone scans play an important role, particularly in identifying occult fractures, and also are very useful in tendinitis and ligamentous injury.

Tips on technique

A three-phase bone scan is always performed. It is important to remember when obtaining the flow and blood pool images that the application of a tourniquet when administering the injection may lead to significant variation in the early perfusion of the limb due to reflex hyperaemia. Early perfusion can also be diffusely affected by disuse and reflex sympathetic dystrophy. To avoid artefacts, it is advisable to insert a butterfly needle into a vein in the contralateral cubital fossa and wait a couple of minutes after removing the tourniquet before injecting. Injection into foot veins is another alternative.

As with all nuclear medicine images, the proximity of the imaged part to the collimator greatly affects the resolution and palmar views are obtained with the hands resting directly on the collimator. Dorsal views are best performed with the hands resting palm down on a table or bed, with the collimator above. This avoids extreme supination when trying to place the dorsum on the collimator, and minimises movement. Simultaneous acquisition of palmar and dorsal views with dual head cameras is suboptimal unless the camera heads can be closely apposed.

Frequently, bony definition is inadequate to resolve individual carpal bones. In some instances, pinhole views may improve resolution and aid in the diagnosis but if bony definition is very poor, pinhole collimation does not help.

Depending on the site of injury, accurate localisation of uptake may be made easier by using some ulnar or radial deviation of the wrist. Sometimes two views, one with deviation and one without, may be helpful. Correlation with an anatomy book or preferably the patient's X-rays will help localise any abnormal uptake.

Extending the field of view to the elbow is essential, as injury at the wrist may be associated with forearm and elbow changes. One way to achieve this is to flex the elbows and rest both arms on the collimator.

Removal of a patient's wrist cast prior to imaging not only reduces attenuation, but also allows proper positioning (Fig. 10.1).

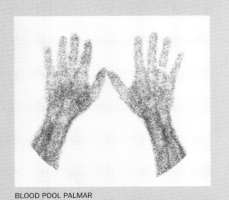
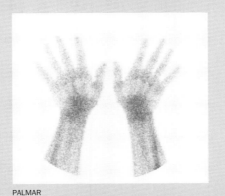
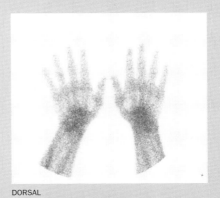

BLOOD POOL PALMAR   PALMAR   DORSAL

Figure 10.1 Standard views. Note that the mild activity in the right third metacarpal bone is a common normal variant.

Fractures (Figs 10.2–10.6)

The most common indication for a bone scan is to assess the wrist for evidence of a fracture following injury. The typical appearance of a fracture is a focal area of increased vascularity on the blood pool images and increased uptake on the delayed images.

A normal plain film with continuing clinical suspicion of a scaphoid fracture is the classic indication for bone scan. Scaphoid fractures make up 70% of all carpal fractures and typically occur after a fall on the outstretched hand. Fractures mostly involve the waist (70%) and can involve the distal pole (20%) and the proximal pole (10%). At the distal pole, with increased uptake, it may be difficult to differentiate a fracture from traumatic synovitis in the scaphotrapezoid joint. This is particularly difficult if the uptake is mild and a pinhole view may be useful. The complications of a fracture in the scaphoid can also be seen on bone scan. Intense activity persisting beyond the time of usual healing suggests delayed union. Early avascular necrosis may show a cold area in the proximal pole of the scaphoid. Later in avascular necrosis the avascular segment will become intensely 'hot' as revascularisation occurs. The authors have seen two cases where the entire scaphoid, rather than the proximal pole, is avascular early after fracture.

Figure 10.2 Fracture of the left scaphoid bone. There is mild focal increase in vascularity and bony uptake across the mid left scaphoid, indicating a recent scaphoid fracture. An X-ray 2 weeks earlier was normal.

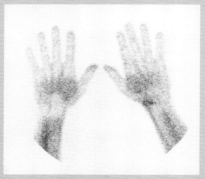

BLOOD POOL PALMAR

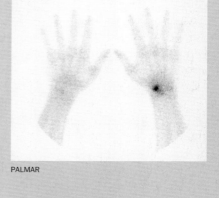

PALMAR

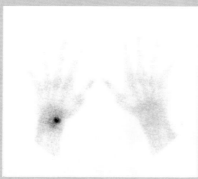

DORSAL

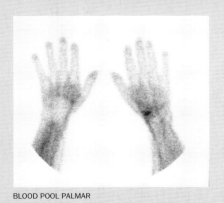

BLOOD POOL PALMAR

PALMAR

Figure 10.3 Left scaphoid fracture. Focal uptake in the left scaphoid on both the blood pool and delayed images indicates recent fracture. The uptake is slightly more intense than in the previous case. There is also arthritis in interphalangeal joints.

PALMAR

Figure 10.4 Recent right scaphoid fracture with intense uptake. Low-grade left scaphoid fracture with mild uptake. These were caused by a fall on the outstretched hands.

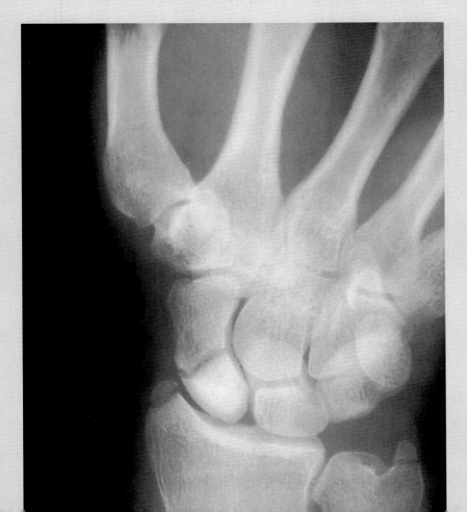

Figure 10.5 Revascularising phase of avascular necrosis in the proximal pole of the right scaphoid. The X-ray shows fracture in the waist of the scaphoid with mild sclerosis in the proximal pole. There are also small fractures in the radial and ulnar styloids. The scan performed 2 months post-injury shows only mild uptake at the fracture sites, with intense uptake in the proximal pole due to revascularisation of post-traumatic avascular necrosis.

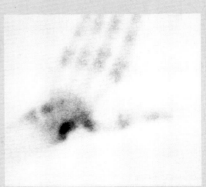

PALMAR

Figure 10.6 Acute right scaphoid fracture with the entire scaphoid being avascular. Plain X-rays at the time of injury were normal. The bone scan performed 3 days later shows increased vascularity in the region of the scaphoid in the blood pool image, but there is absent uptake in the entire scaphoid on the delayed views, indicating avascularity.

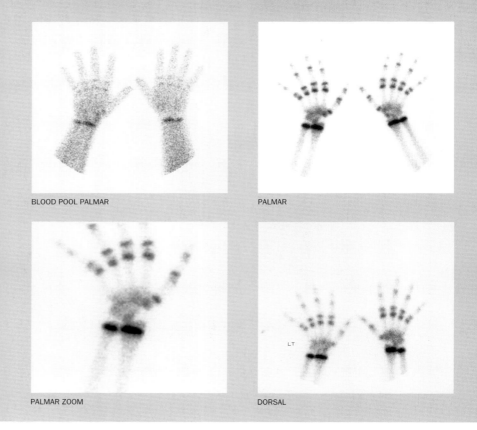

BLOOD POOL PALMAR

PALMAR

PALMAR ZOOM

DORSAL

Fractures of the trapezium can occur as the result of a fall and may be clinically confused with a scaphoid fracture. Fractures of the trapezoid, capitate and lunate are uncommon. When there is increased uptake in the region of the lunate, the differential diagnosis of this appearance would include scapholunate ligament injury, scapholunate or radiocarpal arthritis, avascular necrosis of the lunate or injury to the triangular fibrocartilage complex (Figs 10.7–10.9).

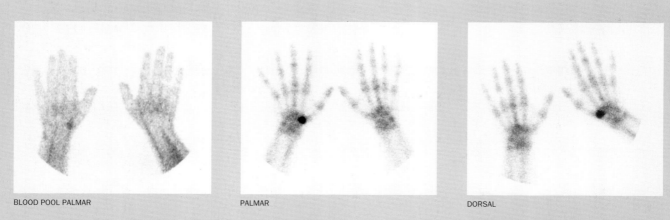

BLOOD POOL PALMAR

PALMAR

DORSAL

Figure 10.7 Fracture of the right trapezium. Care should be taken to accurately localise the uptake and distinguish it from the more common scaphoid fracture or trapezoid fracture.

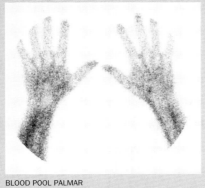

BLOOD POOL PALMAR

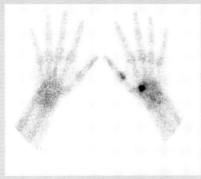

PALMAR

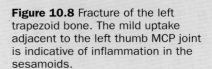

Figure 10.8 Fracture of the left trapezoid bone. The mild uptake adjacent to the left thumb MCP joint is indicative of inflammation in the sesamoids.

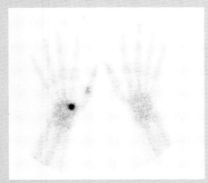

DORSAL

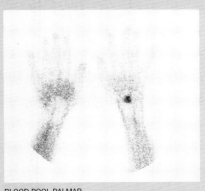

BLOOD POOL PALMAR

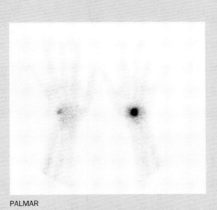

PALMAR

Figure 10.9 Fractured left capitate. There is intense focal blood pool and delayed uptake corresponding to the capitate. While bony definition is poor, knowledge of the anatomy allows localisation to the capitate. Note also low-grade uptake in the right hamate region, indicating a further low-grade fracture.

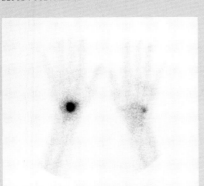

DORSAL

Fractures of the hook of hamate may show a typical localised circular focus of activity on the blood pool and delayed images. This fracture can occur following direct wrist trauma, but can also be seen resulting from bone stress. An additional view with the hand in a vertical position and the ulnar edge of the hand on the collimator ('prayerbook' view) will help demonstrate that the activity is on the palmar side of the carpus (Figs 10.10–10.12).

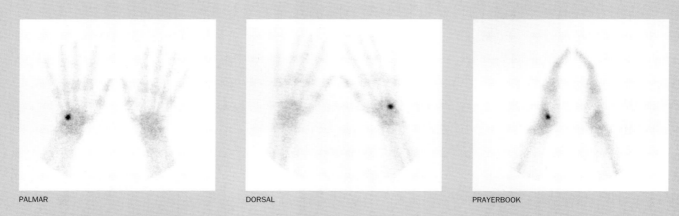

PALMAR　　　　　　　　　　　DORSAL　　　　　　　　　　　PRAYERBOOK

Figure 10.10 Fracture of the right hook of hamate. There is a typical small focus of increased uptake in the right hamate, which the 'prayerbook' view confirms is confined to the palmar side of the wrist.

Figure 10.11 Stress fracture of the hook of hamate in a polo player.

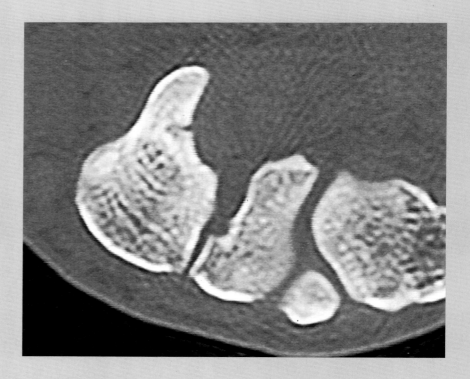

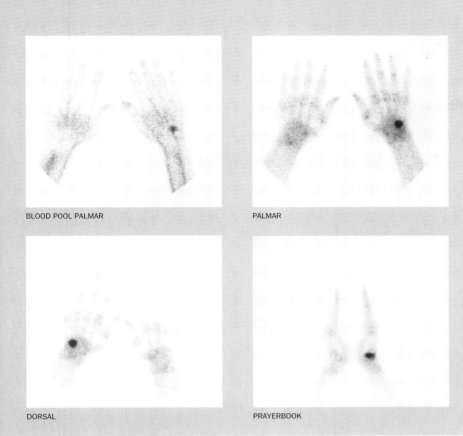

BLOOD POOL PALMAR

PALMAR

DORSAL

PRAYERBOOK

Figure 10.12 Fracture of the left hamate. The blood pool and delayed images show focal intense uptake in the left hamate. Both the palmar and 'prayerbook' views show this is more extensive than in the hook alone, as seen in Figure 10.10.

The pisotriquetral articulation is injured by direct trauma and is stressed in the throwing action and weightbearing activities. As a result, this joint can be the site of bone injury that is difficult to see on plain films. Degenerative changes are often seen in this articulation in relatively young athletes. Mild uptake in the pisotriquetral region is a normal appearance. Greater uptake is seen in arthritis, but more intense uptake, particularly if associated with focal blood pool activity, is most likely indicative of a fracture (Figs 10.13 and 10.14).

Figure 10.13 Advanced degenerative changes in the pisotriquetral articulation in a relatively young wrist. It is likely that the athlete was involved in a throwing or weight-bearing activity.

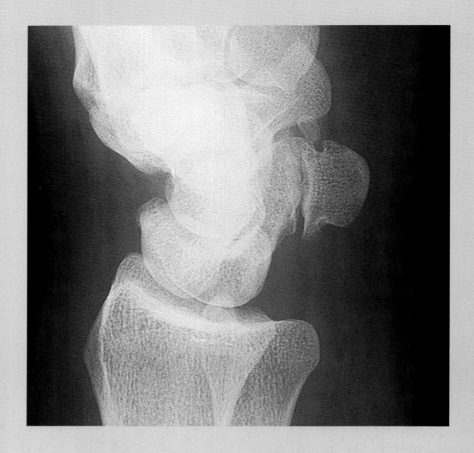

Figure 10.14 Fracture of the right pisotriquetral complex following a fall. The resolution of the bone scan is not good enough to differentiate which of the two bones is fractured.

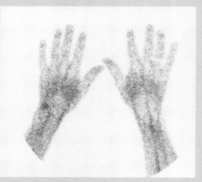

BLOOD POOL PALMAR

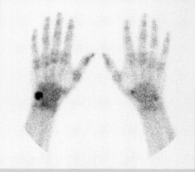

PALMAR

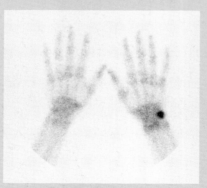

DORSAL

As a general rule, fractures adjacent to a joint in any of the carpal or metacarpal bones may be difficult to distinguish from arthritis, and optimal imaging and careful interpretation are necessary. If the activity is confined to only one side of the joint, then a fracture is most likely.

Fractures of the distal radius and ulna (Figs 10.15–10.23) are very common and many are occult, requiring a bone scan for diagnosis. Disruption of the distal radial growth plate in the immature athlete can be difficult to diagnose on plain films and is best diagnosed on the blood pool images of a bone scan. There is greater vascularity in the growth plate compared to the other arm and relative to the distal ulnar growth plate.

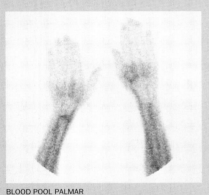

BLOOD POOL PALMAR   PALMAR

Figure 10.15 Fracture across the distal right radius. The early vascularity and delayed uptake are linear across the distal radius, indicating recent fracture.

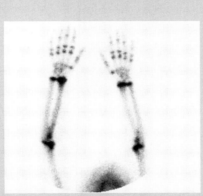

BLOOD POOL PALMAR   PALMAR

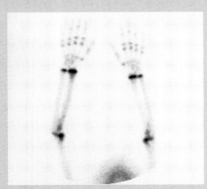

PALMAR LOW INTENSITY

Figure 10.16 Fracture of the distal right radial growth plate. The blood pool image shows increased vascularity across the distal right radial growth plate. This is frequently the most sensitive indicator of bony pathology in children. The delayed images show increased uptake in this growth plate with mild activity in the adjacent metaphysis and to a lesser extent in the right radial shaft. The activity down the shaft represents a reactive response to the fracture at the growth plate. Osteomyelitis is the principal differential diagnosis, although the early vascularity is then usually maximal in the metaphysis rather than the growth plate.

Figure 10.17 Distal right radius and ulna growth plate fractures in a child. The growth plates are a common site of fracture in children, the growth plates being relatively weaker than adjacent bone. The early blood pool image shows the asymmetry in vascularity in the growth plates (left to right). On the delayed views there is increased uptake in both the distal right radial and ulnar growth plates.

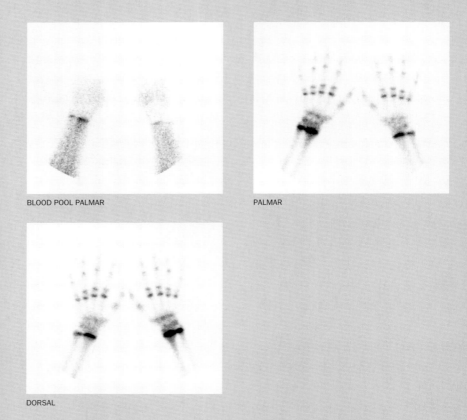

BLOOD POOL PALMAR

PALMAR

DORSAL

Figure 10.18 Localised fracture at the distal right radius adjacent to the radioulnar joint. There is mild vascularity and focal delayed uptake at the ulnar edge of the distal right radius following a recent fall. Note that there is also a subtle increase in uptake in the distal ulna, indicative of low-grade fracture.

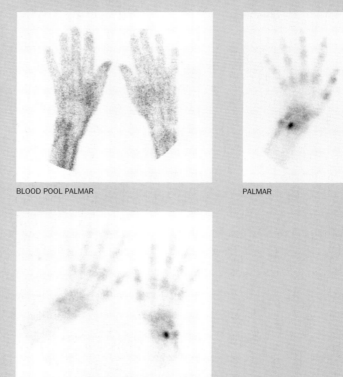

BLOOD POOL PALMAR

PALMAR

DORSAL

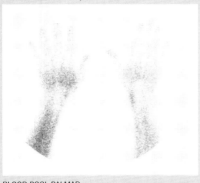

BLOOD POOL PALMAR

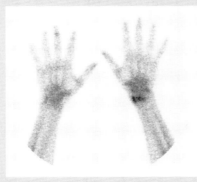

PALMAR

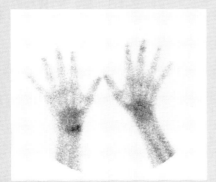

DORSAL

Figure 10.19 Old fracture of the distal left radius with de Quervain's tenosynovitis. The normal vascularity across the distal radius on the blood pool image indicates that the fracture seen at this site on the delayed views is in a later healing stage. There is linear vascularity along the radial edge of the left wrist, with associated delayed uptake along the radial edge of the left radial styloid. This pattern is typical of tenosynovitis.

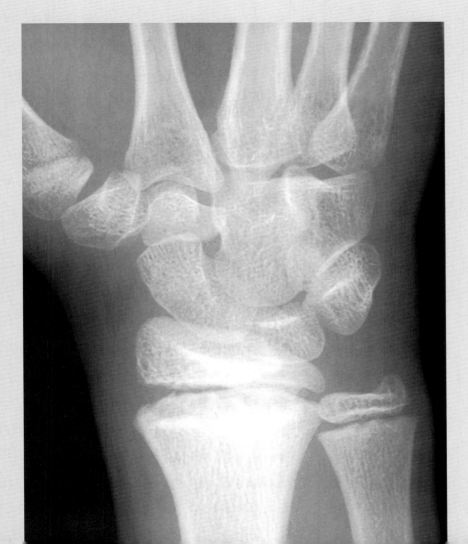

Figure 10.20 'Gymnast wrist' is a stress reaction in the distal radial growth plate due to the weight-bearing use of the wrist in gymnastics.

Figure 10.21 Fracture of the distal right ulna. The increased uptake is predominantly on the radial side of the distal ulna, indicating fracture at this site.

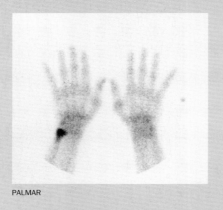 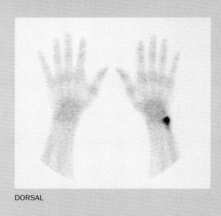

PALMAR   DORSAL

Figure 10.22 Healing fracture of the right ulnar styloid.

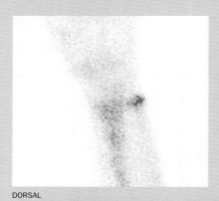

DORSAL

Figure 10.23 Trauma to the right ulna-carpal region. Vascularity and delayed uptake is seen in the region of the triangular fibrocartilage complex and in the pisotriquetral region due to trauma to the complex and adjacent ligaments.

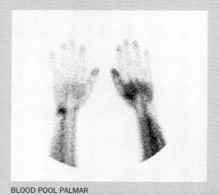 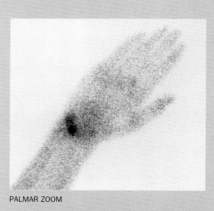

BLOOD POOL PALMAR   PALMAR ZOOM

In the hand, anatomy is simple and bone scans are rarely needed. When diagnosing fractures in the metacarpals (Figs 10.24–10.26), care should be taken not to over-interpret low-grade uptake in the proximal shaft of the third and fourth metacarpals as mild uptake at these sites is a common normal variant.

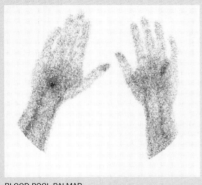

BLOOD POOL PALMAR

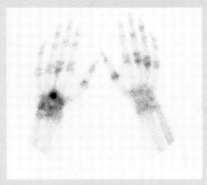

PALMAR

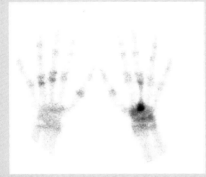

DORSAL

Figure 10.24 Fracture of the base of the right third metacarpal. There is focal vascularity and delayed uptake at the base, with flaring of mild activity along the shaft of the bone. This indicates the primary pathology is in the bone rather than the joint.

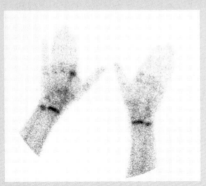

BLOOD POOL PALMAR

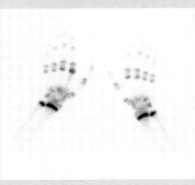

PALMAR

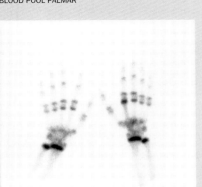

DORSAL

Figure 10.25 Fracture of the growth plate of the head of the right second metacarpal bone. The blood pool image shows the vascularity in the growth plate to be greater than in the adjacent and opposite growth plates. There is also mild activity flaring proximally down the metacarpal shaft on both the blood pool and delayed images.

Figure 10.26 Multiple fractures in the left hand. Recent fractures are present in the head of the left first metacarpal, trapezium and in the hook of the hamate. There is also a small ligament avulsion at the radial side of the head of the left third metacarpal. Multiple injuries like this are frequently observed in contact sports such as rugby.

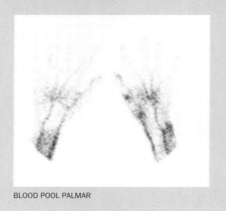

BLOOD POOL PALMAR

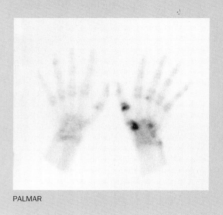

PALMAR

Stress fractures in the hand and wrist are unusual but are occasionally seen involving the distal radial growth plate, the hook of hamate and the pisiform.

Tendinosis (Figs 10.27–10.32)

Overuse may induce pain and tenderness around the tendon or in the tendon sheath. If the diagnosis of tendinosis is considered likely, then the appropriate investigation is ultrasound. However, tendinosis may be observed when scans are undertaken for other causes or the diagnosis is unsuspected. The bone scan may also help confirm the diagnosis and exclude bony pathology simultaneously. De Quervain's tenosynovitis is a common source of pain over the radial styloid. The bone scan shows a line of increased vascularity along the radial edge of the distal forearm and wrist on the flow and blood pool images. The delayed images may be normal or may show low-grade periosteal uptake over the radial styloid. Other sites of tendinitis are less common; however, if linear vascularity is seen, the diagnosis should be considered.

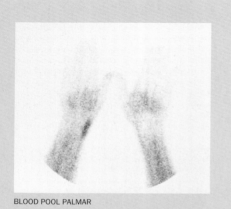

BLOOD POOL PALMAR

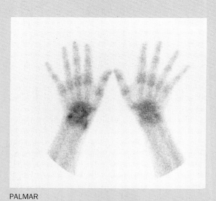

PALMAR

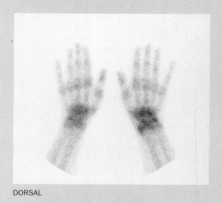

DORSAL

Figure 10.27 Right de Quervain's tenosynovitis. Note that the early vascularity is significantly greater than the delayed bony uptake which is confined to the periosteal edge of the distal radius. There is also mild synovitis throughout the right wrist.

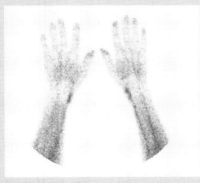

BLOOD POOL PALMAR

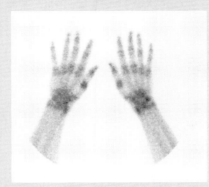

PALMAR

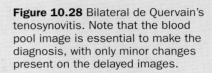

Figure 10.28 Bilateral de Quervain's tenosynovitis. Note that the blood pool image is essential to make the diagnosis, with only minor changes present on the delayed images.

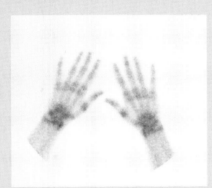

DORSAL

Figure 10.29 Chronic de Quervain's disease. There is soft tissue swelling in the line of the abductor pollicis longus and extensor pollicis brevis, with cortical erosion along the adjacent radial styloid process.

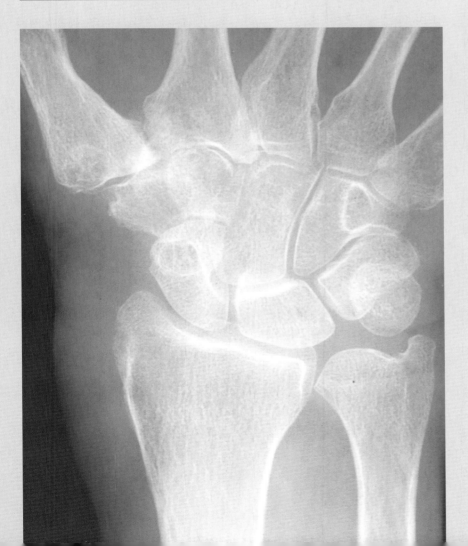

Figure 10.30 Right flexor pollicis longus tenosynovitis. This unusual case occurred in an office worker performing repetitive thumb flexion removing 'bulldog' clips from files. Note the linear increase in vascularity in the line of the flexor pollicis longus tendon in the early view. Foci of uptake in the hook of hamate and base of the third metacarpal are most likely due to stress fractures. (Images courtesy of Dr D McHarg and Dr J Burke.)

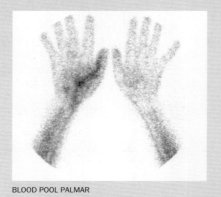
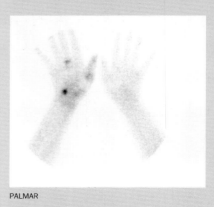

BLOOD POOL PALMAR

PALMAR

Figure 10.31 Tendinopathy involving the right flexor carpi radialis is well demonstrated by ultrasound.

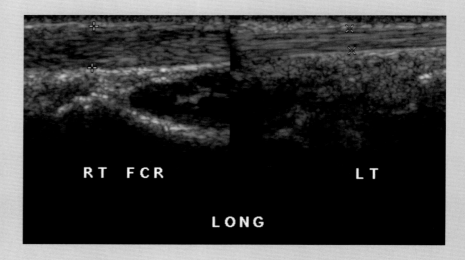

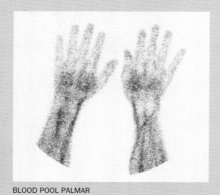
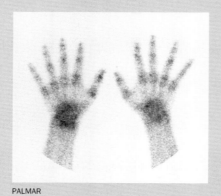
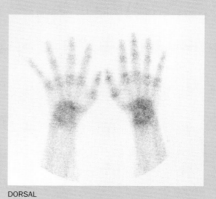

BLOOD POOL PALMAR

PALMAR

DORSAL

Figure 10.32 Extensor tendinosis of the right wrist due to repetitive flexion and extension wrist movements in a house painter. Note the linear increase in blood pool in the distal right forearm, with no focal increase in uptake on the delayed images.

Synovitis/osteoarthritis (Figs 10.33–10.34)

Traumatic synovitis following injury is a common occurrence. In the wrist this will frequently involve the entire carpal region, while elsewhere in the hand it may be confined to only a single joint or adjacent joints. It may be present in conjunction with other bony injuries or may be the only evidence of trauma. The bone scan typically shows a diffuse increase in vascularity throughout the joint. There is mild to moderate diffusely increased uptake on the delayed views.

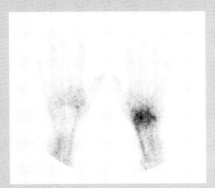

BLOOD POOL PALMAR

PALMAR

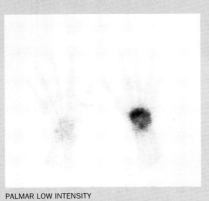

PALMAR LOW INTENSITY

Figure 10.33 Traumatic synovitis in the left wrist. There is a diffuse increase in blood pool activity and intense delayed uptake throughout the carpal region. On the less intense display, there is greater uptake at the carpo-metacarpal junction. This injury is similar to the Lisfranc's fracture dislocation in the foot.

Osteoarthritis is a common finding on bone scans and usually shows a more focal pattern of uptake. Careful attention to the distribution of uptake and correlation with the clinical history is important to differentiate focal arthritic uptake from bony trauma. This can be particularly difficult in osteochondral fractures where both fracture and synovitis may be present. While focal vascularity is often a guide to bony trauma, osteoarthritis can also have an increased blood flow.

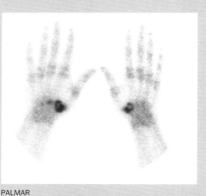 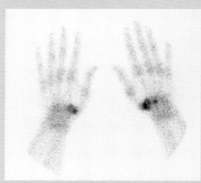

Figure 10.34 Osteoarthritis in the first metacarpal-trapezium-trapezoid joint complex bilaterally. This is a very common site of arthritis. Care should be taken to localise the uptake accurately to distinguish joint from bone pathology.

PALMAR

DORSAL

Ligament injuries (Figs 10.35–10.37)

Following trauma, a ligamentous avulsion injury will give a bone scan appearance of a very small focal area of increased uptake at the avulsion site. This may represent a small chip fracture. The activity is greatest on the delayed image although a mild focal increase in vascularity may also be seen on the blood pool image. The commoner sites of ligamentous insertion injury include the scapholunate and lunotriquetral articulations, the posterior tubercle of the triquetrum, the medial aspect of the base of the first proximal phalanx and the radial edge of the scaphoid.

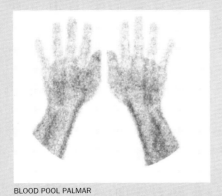

BLOOD POOL PALMAR

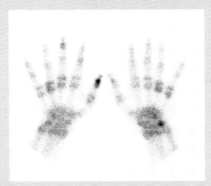

PALMAR

Figure 10.35 Right thumb small avulsion fracture at the base of the distal phalanx. There is also left pisotriquetral arthritis. Note that the dorsal view of the left hand is positioned with radial deviation of the wrist, aiding in localisation of the pisotriquetral pathology.

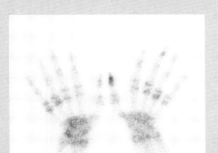

DORSAL

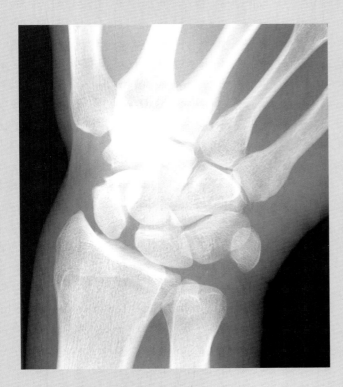

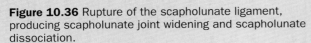

Figure 10.36 Rupture of the scapholunate ligament, producing scapholunate joint widening and scapholunate dissociation.

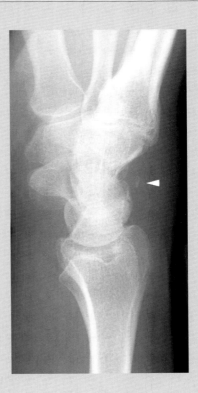

Figure 10.37 Avulsion of the dorsal radiocarpal ligament from the posterior tubercle of the triquetrum (arrow).

Other conditions (Figs 10.38 and 10.39)

Reflex sympathetic dystrophy can occur in the hand and wrist following shoulder, arm or hand injury. This injury may not be particularly severe and is often associated with prolonged disuse. A number of patterns of activity have been described on bone scan and different patterns may occur at different stages of the disease. The typical appearance is of diffusely increased blood flow throughout the distal limb on the blood pool images, and periarticular uptake in the wrist and fingers on the delayed images. Reduced blood flow and uptake have also been described. It can be difficult to determine whether the bone scan changes are purely due to prolonged disuse or to reflex sympathetic dystrophy.

Figure 10.38 Reflex sympathetic dystrophy of the right wrist and hand secondary to a healed fracture of the distal radius. The blood pool image shows mild diffusely increased vascularity throughout the right wrist and hand compared to the left. On delayed views there is increased uptake in the right wrist and hand, particularly in a periarticular distribution. While this is a common appearance of reflex sympathetic dystrophy, other patterns of increased or reduced vascularity and bony uptake may be seen.

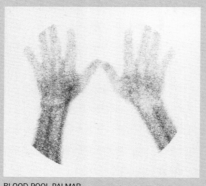

BLOOD POOL PALMAR

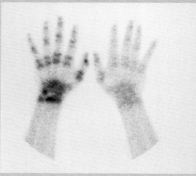

PALMAR

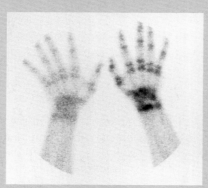

DORSAL

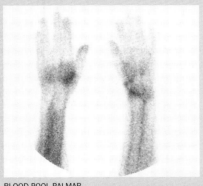

BLOOD POOL PALMAR

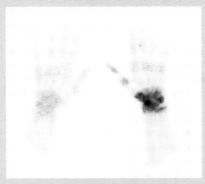

PALMAR

Figure 10.39 Regional reflex sympathetic dystrophy of the left wrist secondary to a previous scaphoid fracture. There is a diffuse increase in vascularity and bony uptake in the left carpal bones and in a periarticular distribution in the left thumb. The scan appearances of regional reflex sympathetic dystrophy and regional osteoporosis are similar and are probably both parts of the same pathophysiological process of autonomic dysfunction.

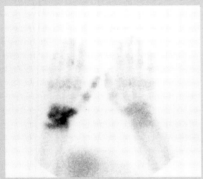

DORSAL

Avascular necrosis of the lunate is rarely imaged in the initial 'cold' phase and is usually seen in the later 'hot' phase with focal uptake throughout the lunate on both the early and delayed views. Avascular necrosis of the scaphoid is a post-traumatic complication and will show reduced uptake in the proximal pole in the early 'cold' stage, progressing to increased uptake with revascularisation.

Ulnar variance is the relative inequality in the length of the ulna compared with the radius. Normally, the load is shared between the radius and ulna in an 80:20 per cent ratio. With ulna lengthening (ulna plus variance), the ulnar load is increased and ulnar impingement (ulnar abutment syndrome) or damage to the triangular fibrocartilage complex can occur. The condition is diagnosed on plain X-ray, but the bone scan may confirm bony change at the abutment sites. Ulna shortening (ulna minus variance) has been associated with carpal instability and avascular necrosis of the lunate (Figs 10.40 and 10.41).

Figure 10.40 Left ulnar impingement. There is uptake in both the ulnar styloid and in the pisotriquetral region. This appearance is seen in ulna plus variance and is also termed 'ulnar abutment syndrome'.

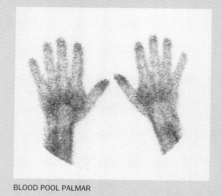

BLOOD POOL PALMAR

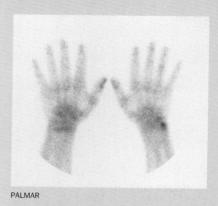

PALMAR

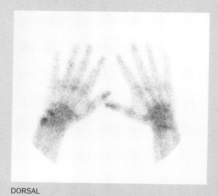

DORSAL

Figure 10.41 Avascular necrosis of the lunate is commonly associated with ulna minus variance.

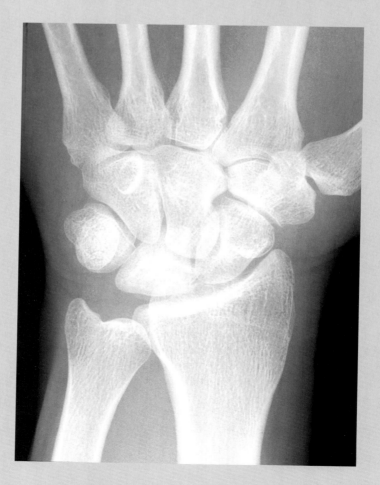

Bibliography

Chidgey, LK, Chronic wrist pain, *Orthopedic Clinics of North America* 23: 1992, pp 49–64

Cooney, WP, Dobyns, JH, Linscheid, RL, Fractures of the scaphoid: a rational approach to management, *Clin Orthop* 14: 1980, pp 90–7

Desai, A, Intenzo, C, The 'tourniquet effect', *J Nucl Med* 25: 1984, pp 697–9

Hawkes, DJ, Robinson, L, Crossman, JF, Sayman, HB, Mistry, R, Maisey, MN, Spencer, JD, Registration & display of the combined bone scan & radiograph in the diagnosis & management of wrist injuries, *Eur J Nucl Med* 18: 1991, pp 752–6

Holder, LE, Mackinnon, SE, Reflex sympathetic dystrophy in the hands: clinical and scintigraphic criteria, *Radiology* 152: 1984, pp 517–22

Holder, LE, Mulligan, ME, Gillespie, TE, Diagnosis of scaphoid fractures: The role of Nuclear Medicine. Editorial, *J Nucl Med* 36: 1995, pp 48–50

Miller, JH, Osterkamp, JA, Scintigraphy in acute plastic bowing of the forearm, *Radiology* 142: 1982, p 742

Palmer, AK, Glisson, RR, Werner, FW, Ulnar Variance determination *J Hand Surg* 7: 1982, pp 376–9

Patel, N, Collier, BD, Carrera, GF, Hanel, DP, Sanger, JR, Matloub, AS, Hackbarth, DA, Krasnow, AZ, Hellman, RS, Isitman, AT, High resolution bone scintigraphy of the adult wrist, *Clin Nucl Med* 17: 1992, pp 449–53

Stark, HH, Jobe, FW, Boyes, JH, Fracture of the hook of the hamate in athletes, *J Bone Joint Surg* [Am] 59: 1977, pp 575–82

Tiel-van Buul, MMC, Broekhurzen, TH, Van Beek, EJ, Which strategy for the diagnostic management of suspected scaphoid fracture? A cost effective analysis, *J Nucl Med* 35: 1994, pp 45–8

Vande Streek, P, Carretta, RF, Weiland, FL, Shelton, DK, Upper extremity radionuclide bone imaging: The wrist & hand, *Semin Nucl Med* 28: 1998, pp 14–24

Index

Page numbers in **bold** print refer to main entries.
Page numbers in *italics* refer to illustrations.